So, You Need to Go to the Doctor?

How to get the medical care you need & deserve

Charles Lebowitz MD, FACP
Fellow of the American College of Physicians

Illustrations, cover & page design ©2005 Chris Williams

authorHOUSE™

1663 Liberty Drive, Suite 200
Bloomington, Indiana 47403
(800) 839-8640
www.AuthorHouse.com

First published by AuthorHouse 05/12/05

ISBN: 1-4208-5317-1 (sc)
ISBN: 1-4208-5316-3 (dj)

Printed in the United States of America
Bloomington, Indiana

This book is printed on acid-free paper.

Contents

Foreword

Patient: *"Doc, if I don't eat rich foods or red meats, if I don't smoke cigarettes or drink alcohol, and if I don't cavort with wild women, will I live longer?"*
Doctor: *After thinking a second, "No, it will only seem longer."* (Author Unknown)

This book will help you to obtain proper medical care. Everybody deserves to receive the highest quality of medical care. There is a section on obtaining the correct health insurance. This is extremely important, because without health insurance you will not have access to proper medical treatment. This is simply a reality in today's society. I have also shared with you the evaluation, diagnosis and treatment of many different medical problems. This will include evaluation and treatment of chest pain and heart disease. There are also sections on alcoholism and drug abuse, which is so prevalent in our society. You will also learn about the history of medical treatment of HIV and other sexually transmitted diseases. There is even a section on how to find the right doctor and how to be certain that a particular Physician is correct for you.

All of the topics in this book will be relevant for obtaining the best medical care possible.

I hope you enjoy reading this book. Please use this book as a guide to staying healthy and receiving proper medical care.

Dedication

I dedicate this book to my entire family, especially my wife, Sharon. She has been my inspiration and soul mate, since the first day we met. In addition, she never complained when she had to listen to me talk about writing a book, for the last year. She has always stood by me and motivated me to pursue my dreams.

I want to thank my parents for always supporting me, in all of my endeavors. My father still thinks of me as his little boy. My mother, I know, is looking from the heavens at all of us, and is so proud. She still gives me strength and security. My brothers Allan and Fred, and sister Helen, have always believed in me and held me to a higher standard. They always encouraged me to be the best I could be. When times were tough, they were always there for me. They know what I mean.

Finally, I want to thank my children, Ilisa and Randy. They are the greatest gifts that a person could ever have. I am so proud of them. They have grown into such wonderful adults and are so honorable and forthright. They have a fantastic future ahead of them. I love them so much and have enjoyed every second that I have spent with them.

Oh - I almost forgot - to my special buddies - Jacques, Boychik, and Jake - my dogs, for their unconditional love and for always being happy and making me feel good. They always keep the world in its proper perspective, and help me to enjoy life's simple things.

1 | Heart Disease

I have a number of exam rooms in my office. Patients are examined first by a nurse and have their vital signs (blood pressure, pulse, and temperature) taken. They also tell the nurse what their problem is, and this is written into the chart. Then, when I come into the exam room, the patient will be ready for me to examine. This is how it was on a Wednesday morning, in August. The heat of the day was evident early in our Florida morning. The humidity was high as was the temperature. Inside the office, the air conditioner was on full blast and it wasn't even 9:00 am. Cold air was streaming from the air conditioner vents. As I entered the next exam room, Mr. Harrison was on the exam table. He was with his wife in the room and she had a worried look on her face. Sometimes, the spouse can reveal more than the patient. He was a Marine and 43 years old. He was obviously still in good shape. He participated in the Marines' physical conditioning programs on a regular basis. He had "muscles on his muscles." He had a buzz haircut and his shirt was off. There were beads of sweat on his hair and dripping off his face and he said, "Doc - you have to turn the air up!" The room that he was in was really quite cold and I wondered why he was so hot and sweaty. I asked him "What's doing? What brought you in today?" He replied, " My left shoulder is hurting. It's been going off and on for a week and not getting any better. Sometimes, I feel a tingle in my jaw. I am also feeling a little dizzy." He told me that he went to the Marine doctor and was given some anti-inflammatory medicines and they haven't helped. I asked him about the pain. "Does it hurt when you move your arm or is the pain constant?" He replied, "Moving my arm doesn't make it any worse. It seems to get bad when I walk or run. " He described the area that was causing him pain. He said, " The pain is in my shoulder area and I really can't say where the pain is exactly. It also seems to go into my left neck and my jaw. Maybe it's a toothache?"

At that point, I started to become suspicious that something other than a strained shoulder was happening. I peeked my head out of the door and asked my nurse to perform an EKG (electrocardiogram). While the nurse was doing this procedure, I was able to talk to the patient and his wife. I asked, "Do you still smoke cigarettes?" I knew that he did, I was able to smell tobacco on his body. I also knew that he had high blood pressure and didn't like to take his medications.

He viewed having high blood pressure as a weakness. He wasn't the type of man to have any weaknesses. I asked his wife about his diet. She stated, "He likes his meat and potatoes - he needs to be strong".

His family history didn't help me very much. His father had died in a military training accident at a young age. His mother was still alive, but he didn't know about any of her medical problems. He was an only child. He and his wife had 4 children and they were all in school today. I looked at the EKG. I was able to see it upside down as it came out of the machine. Even looking at it from that viewpoint, I was able to see it wasn't normal. My suspicions were confirmed. The EKG showed elevations of the ST segments (figures 1-a and 1-b). This is part of the EKG waveform that would show decreased blood flow to a particular area of the heart. The segment of this EKG was for the front of the heart. We call this pattern of waveforms "tombstones", because it looks like a grave marker, as well as its high potential for death. He then told me, "Doc, the pain is getting a little worse. It feels like my whole left arm is being squeezed in a vise." He was sweating and appeared a little ashen and short of breath. I immediately gave him a nitroglycerin under his tongue and placed him on oxygen through a tube into his nose. I signaled for one of the nurses to call 911 and to arrange for emergency transport to the hospital. I also spoke to an invasive cardiologist to have him brought directly to the catheterization laboratory. His wife was really concerned. She asked me "Are you sure? How could this be - he is so strong. It's just his shoulder and that should be looked at." I tried to explain to the patient and his wife that I believed that he was having a heart attack and this needed to be taken care of right away. What happened next was almost unbelievable. They actually seemed relieved. They understood that something serious was happening to him. However, they were glad to have the situation finally taken care of. They were happy that they finally had a diagnosis and that they would receive treatment. I think that both of them strongly suspected that the problem was his heart. The Emergency Medical Services (EMS) arrived, and they placed him on a stretcher, and took him off to the hospital. I gave him an aspirin and a Plavix just before he left the office. I also gave him another nitroglycerin and a lot of his pain subsided. He was brought directly to the hospital, where an invasive cardiology team was awaiting his arrival.

normal EKG

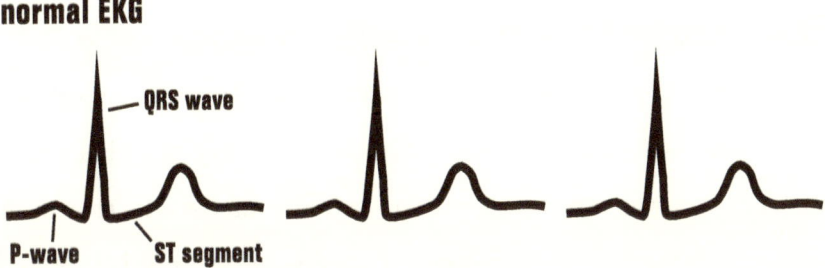

Fig. 1-a. Electrocardiogram - normal waves. There are the following waves on an EKG:

P-wave - contraction of the atria (upper chambers)

QRS - wave - contraction of the ventricles (lower chambers)

S-T segment - where you look to see if the patient is having a heart attack - if it is elevated, that means there is a decreased blood supply to the heart from an occluded coronary artery. This S-T segment is flat.

abnormal EKG

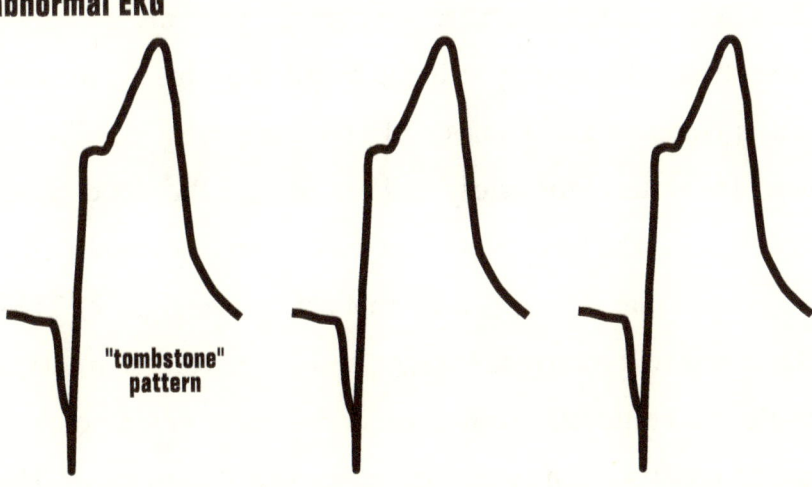

Fig. 1-b. Electrocardiogram of a person with a heart attack - see "tombstone pattern." The S-T segment is elevated and this patient is having a heart attack. The configuration of the S-T segment looks like a tombstone. A patient with this EKG pattern is in a lot of danger.

So what happened to this patient? How can someone that is so young and apparently healthy have a problem with his heart? That's actually easy to understand. It wasn't his whole heart that was the problem, only the coronary arteries (fig. 1-c). The arteries that run on the outside of the heart are the coronary arteries. At least one artery was occluded (blocked) (fig. 1-d). These are the very arteries that feed the heart its blood supply. It would be logical to question why the heart needs these arteries, since it's pumping all of the body's blood through its chambers. The heart is basically a big muscle. The arteries feed the muscle with its blood supply. The muscles of the heart don't get their blood supply from the blood in the chambers. That blood is being pumped to the rest of the body. The arteries in the heart are very small. They are extremely susceptible to becoming occluded by **plaque**. This is a material that is composed of cholesterol and other fats. It builds up along the walls of the artery and can occlude the blood vessel. By occluding the blood vessel, no blood can be transported to the muscle that is supplied by that artery (see fig. 1-c). Thus, the muscle will receive no oxygen and it can result in injury or death of that muscle. In the case of the heart, when no blood can be received in a particular area, pain will develop. This pain is called **angina pectoris**. The pain will increase when the person is exercising or walking. That is because the heart is pumping harder and faster and needs even more blood than while the person is at rest.

What are the **signs and symptoms** of CAD (coronary artery disease)? CAD develops gradually. At first, the coronary arteries accumulate some fatty plaque. The plaque eventually increases in size and hardens as it becomes calcified. This means that less blood can go through the blood vessel, that feeds the heart muscle. When the heart is deprived of blood flow and oxygen, the person will develop pain. Usually the pain is described as tightness in the chest. It sometimes causes pain in the arms, mainly the left arm. The patient usually describes shortness of breath and sweating. Commonly, angina will cause the patient to be nauseated. Sometimes, all of these symptoms will be described, and at other times, there may be atypical symptoms. For example, my patient, Mr. Harrison only had pain in the shoulder and shortness of breath. He felt warm and sweaty (diaphoresis). He had no chest pain at all. At first, the patient will have anginal (chest pain from the heart) pain only with exertion. As the blockage of the coronary artery increases in size, the patient may progress to having **pain at rest**. This is called **unstable angina** and is a very dangerous situation.

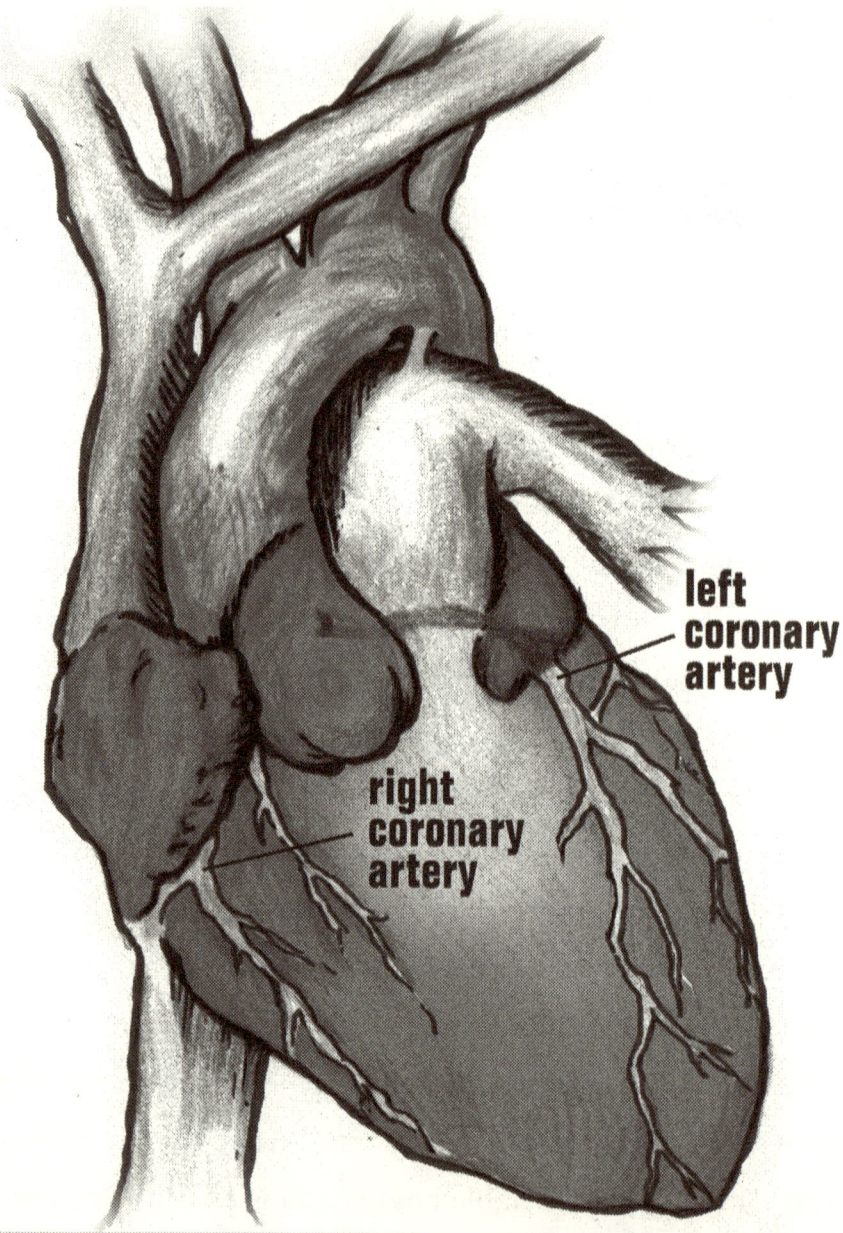

Fig. 1-c. The normal heart and the coronary arteries. These arteries are on the outside of the heart, and supply its blood (and thus oxygen).

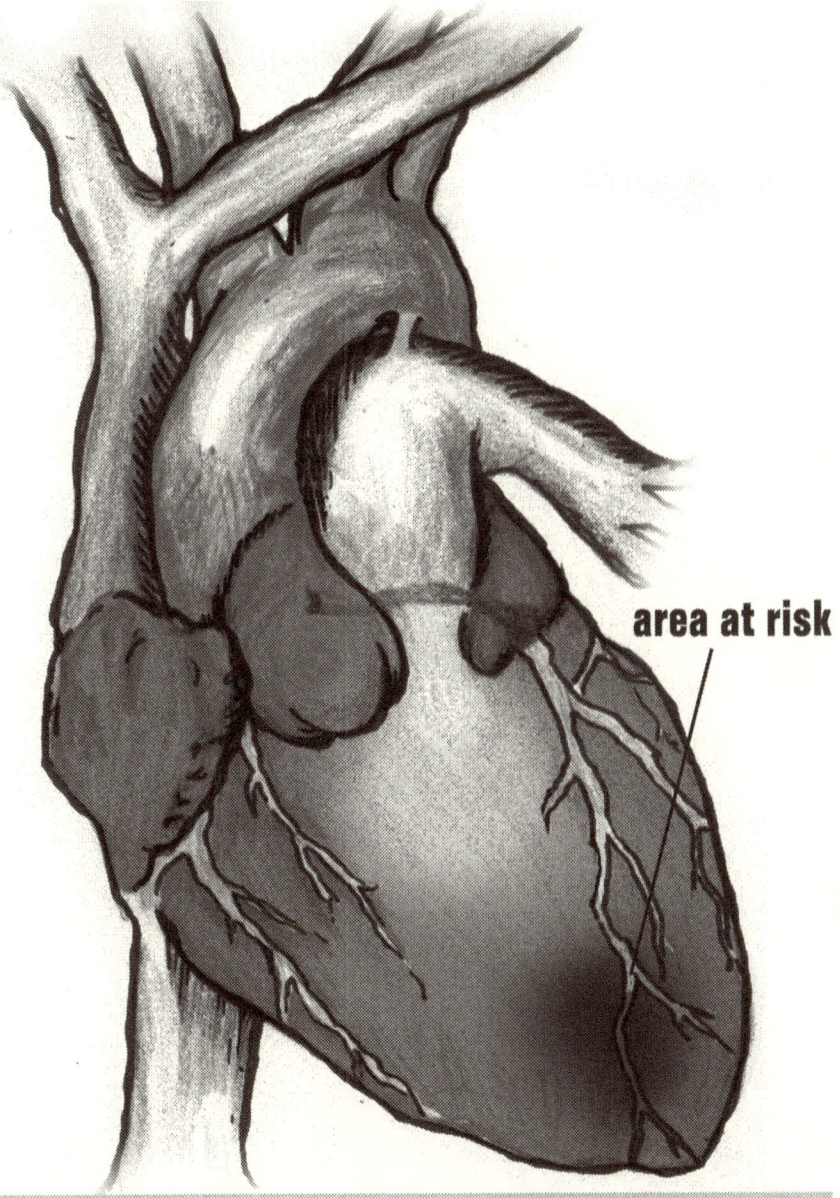

area at risk

Fig. 1-d. An artery occluded by plaque and clot. When an artery is occluded, no blood flow can pass the plaque. In the case of a sudden heart attack, the plaque will get a crack in it. The blood clot will form in the plaque and completely block the artery. No blood will be able to get past the clot. We use Aspirin to prevent this clot from forming.

2 | Diagnosis: Coronary Artery Disease

Walking is the best possible exercise. Habituate yourself to walk very far."
Thomas Jefferson (1743 - 1826)

The diagnosis of coronary artery disease (CAD) can be either very obvious or at times elusive. Special testing can be required to determine the cause of someone's chest pain or to see if someone has underlying coronary artery disease. The most common way that a doctor will determine if chest pain is due to coronary artery disease is by the symptoms. Doctors frequently ask questions about the chest pain. "Where is it located?" is the first question that should be asked. Most commonly, the chest pain of a heart attack or coronary artery disease is located to the left of the sternum (chest- wall) and will frequently travel up to the left side of the neck and down the left arm. Usually, the chest pain is described as squeezing or tightness around the chest area. Frequently, patients will say "something heavy is sitting on my chest." In addition, patients will usually use a "closed fist" sign. That means that when they describe the chest pain they are tightening their fist to describe the type of sensation that they are feeling, inside of their chest. The chest pain is frequently associated with shortness of breath or inability to catch one's breath. There is frequently nausea, sometimes vomiting, and most commonly sweating (called diaphoresis in medical terminology).

Mr. Harrison had many of these symptoms. The cause of his chest pain could have been diagnosed on the basis of the symptoms alone. He clearly had coronary artery disease based on the physical characteristics of his pain and the associated symptoms that accompanied the pain, i.e. shortness of breath, nausea, and the radiation of the pain down his left arm.

The first thing that a Physician will do when evaluating someone's chest pain, is a physical examination. You cannot conclusively tell that a patient is having a heart attack by the physical examination. However, you can rule out other causes of chest pain such as a collapsed lung (pneumothorax) or pericarditis. In addition, if the patient is having severe chest wall pain (costochondritis), that can be elucidated by simply pressing on the chest wall. The patient will have increased pain with the doctor pressing on the chest wall, if the pain is from inflamed ribs. There is usually a muscle strain or inflammation of the ribs or breastbone that can cause severe chest pain. There are many other diseases that can simulate a heart attack such as: a pulmonary embolism (blood clot to the lungs), aortic dissection (think John Ritter), or even simple reflux of acid from the stomach into the food pipe (esophagus). All of these conditions can cause chest pain that mimics a heart attack.

The first test that a Physician will do to determine the cause of chest pain is an electrocardiogram (EKG). This test can help doctors diagnose a heart attack, as well as other heart problems. The electrocardiogram records the electrical activity of the patient's heart through electrodes attached to the skin. The electrocardiogram will usually print out from a print recorder. The Physician can get an electrocardiogram within minutes of the patient arriving in the office. If the patient is having a heart attack, this can usually be seen as changes on the electrocardiogram. The electrocardiogram can show that either a heart attack has occurred in the past, or there is one in progress. Also, the electrocardiogram can show the Physician the heart rate, the heart rhythm, and can frequently even tell the Physician the size of the heart. If there is an electrolyte abnormality (Sodium, Calcium and Potassium), this can be seen on the EKG.

If the pain is severe, or the diagnosis is uncertain, the patient should be hospitalized. The next test that should be done would be a blood test. When a patient is having damage to the heart from decreased blood flow through the arteries, the heart muscle becomes damaged. When the heart muscle becomes damaged, certain enzymes that normally reside within the heart muscle, are released into the bloodstream. Damage to the heart cells from a heart attack can cause these enzymes to leak into the blood stream. The two most common blood tests that are evaluated at this time are the CPK, or creatinine phosphokinase, and the Troponin-1. Evaluation of these blood tests can certainly aid in the diagnosis of an acute heart attack or myocardial infarction. However, these tests are usually not available in doctor's offices and can take some time to come back from a laboratory. Creatinine phosphokinase is also found in the brain, heart, and skeletal muscle. Levels of this will rise within 4-6 hours of a heart attack and peak in 18-24 hours. That is why this test is usually repeated during a patient's stay in the hospital, as the initial test may be normal, even though the patient is having a heart attack. It takes a certain amount of time for the levels of CPK to rise within the bloodstream. Troponin is a protein that helps your heart muscle contract. Troponin levels increase right away after a heart attack and remain elevated for up to two weeks. It is highly specific and sensitive to heart tissue injury. This is the blood test most commonly used as an indicator of an acute heart attack.

If a patient had chest pain and the electrocardiogram and blood tests are all negative for an acute heart attack, a

Physician may then request a stress test. A stress test is a dynamic test that helps measure the blood flow to the heart. An exercise stress test is where a patient walks on a treadmill and the electrocardiogram is monitored. A Physician will attempt to see if the chest pain can be reproduced by exercise. Also, the electrocardiogram is monitored during a stress test. If there is decreased blood flow through the coronary arteries, this will be shown in the electrocardiogram pattern. There will be specific changes in the electrocardiogram for a patient with coronary artery disease.

Sometimes, the results of the stress test are not definitive and a nuclear stress test needs to be performed. This is also called a perfusion stress test. In this test, you receive an injection of radioactive materials, usually Thallium. You get the injection when you reach your maximum level of exercise. Then images of the heart are made shortly after exercise and again a few hours later. This test shows how well blood flows into the heart muscle and can indicate the presence of coronary artery disease. The nuclear stress test is much more sensitive than just a regular exercise stress test. However, it is much more complicated and certainly more expensive.

Generally, the best test to determine if a patient has blocked coronary arteries is the coronary artery catheterization, or cardiac angiogram (fig. 1-d). This test helps doctors identify individual arteries to your heart that may be narrowed or blocked. What happens is that through a blood vessel in the groin, the femoral artery, a catheter, or tube, is passed up to the heart into the coronary arteries. A liquid dye is injected into the arteries of the heart through this catheter. As the dye fills the arteries, X-rays are taken of the heart. The Physician can then see immediately if the arteries are occluded. This is by far the best test to determine if someone's arteries are occluded. However, of course, this test requires the patient to be in a hospital and is what is called an invasive test, i.e., the test requires a catheter to be passed up to the heart through a large vessel in the groin area. It also requires the patient to have an injection of dye, for which there can be an allergic reaction or a complication. However, since this test is so frequently performed, advances have been made and fewer people have major side effects to the test.

The best thing about a coronary angiogram is that if an artery is found occluded, it could be opened by **coronary angioplasty** (fig. 2-a). This is a procedure to dilate a blocked artery. This procedure is also known as coronary artery balloon dilation, balloon angioplasty, or PTCA. During the angioplasty, a tiny balloon is threaded through a blood vessel in your groin up into a coronary artery. This is done to widen an area that has become blocked with plaque. What happens is that a catheter is passed up to the arteries in the heart. The artery that is found to be blocked has the catheter passed into it. The end of the catheter has a tiny balloon at the end, which is filled with air, and the plaque that is in the arteries is crushed, and the area that has become blocked is now open. After the angioplasty, it is standard now to place a small wire mesh tube (**stent**) inside the heart artery where the blockage was. The stent holds the artery open more widely and reduces the likelihood that the artery will re-narrow in the same spot. The stents are like little meshes or small little cages. Recently, the stents have been coated with a certain drug, or medication, that will help prevent this area of the artery from becoming re-occluded, or re-blocked. This is called a **drug-eluting stent**.

After examining Mr. Harrison, we performed an electrocardiogram. This clearly showed that he was having a heart attack. I really did not need any more information to tell me what we needed to do. He was taken by ambulance to the hospital. I gave him some aspirin to help keep the arteries open. He was also given nitroglycerin to relieve his chest pain. His chest pain subsided before the ambulance came. His electrocardiogram also reverted to normal, after we gave him a few nitroglycerin tablets. He told me he felt better and actually wanted to go home. This was very typical Marine mentality. He was macho and nothing could harm him. Unfortunately, a very small artery that supplied his heart with blood flow and thus oxygen was occluded. This artery had to be opened, by an angioplasty.

I contacted one of the cardiologists and this patient was brought directly to the cardiac catheterization laboratory at our hospital. He underwent an angiogram, which revealed that he had an occluded left anterior descending artery. He subsequently underwent an angioplasty, which opened up the artery. He then had a stent placed into the artery (fig. 2-b). Hopefully this will keep the artery open forever.

Mr. Harrison did very well after his procedure. But what is his prognosis? In other words, will he not have any further coronary artery occlusions? He needed to reduce his risk factors for coronary artery disease. Will he continue to have blocked arteries, or will he stay healthy?

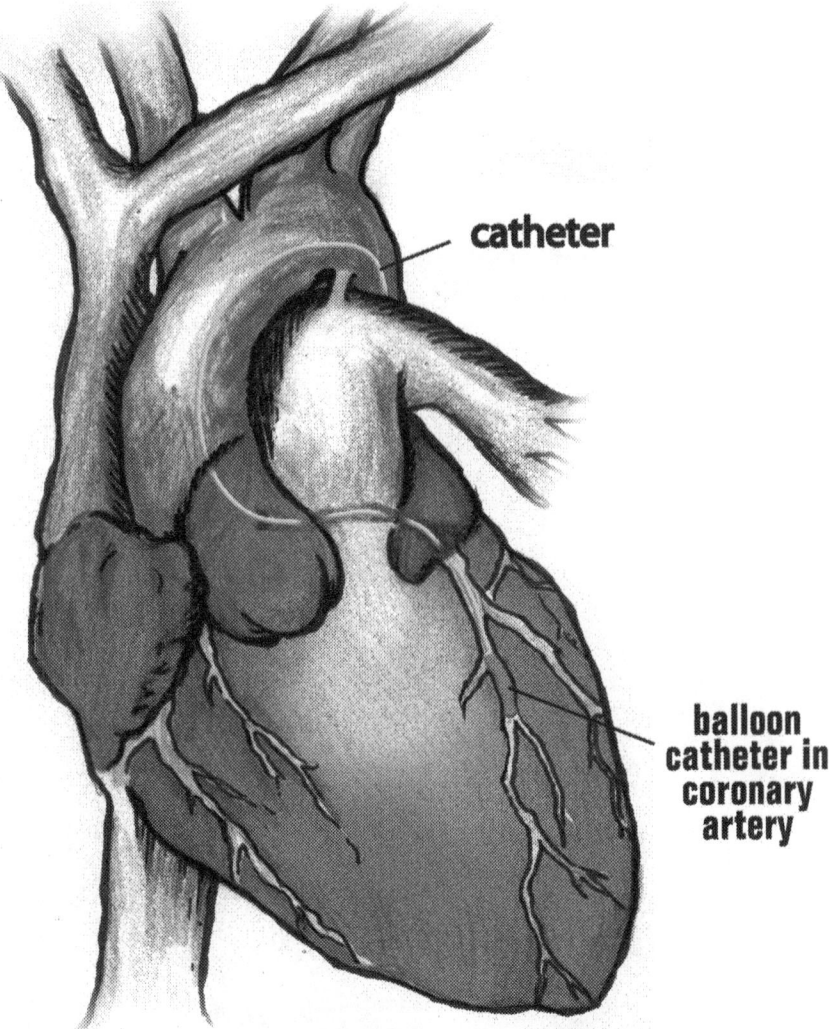

Fig. 2-a. Coronary angioplasty - a balloon is passed into the coronary artery and the blockage is crushed. This opens the artery to blood flow. A stent is then inserted to keep the artery open.

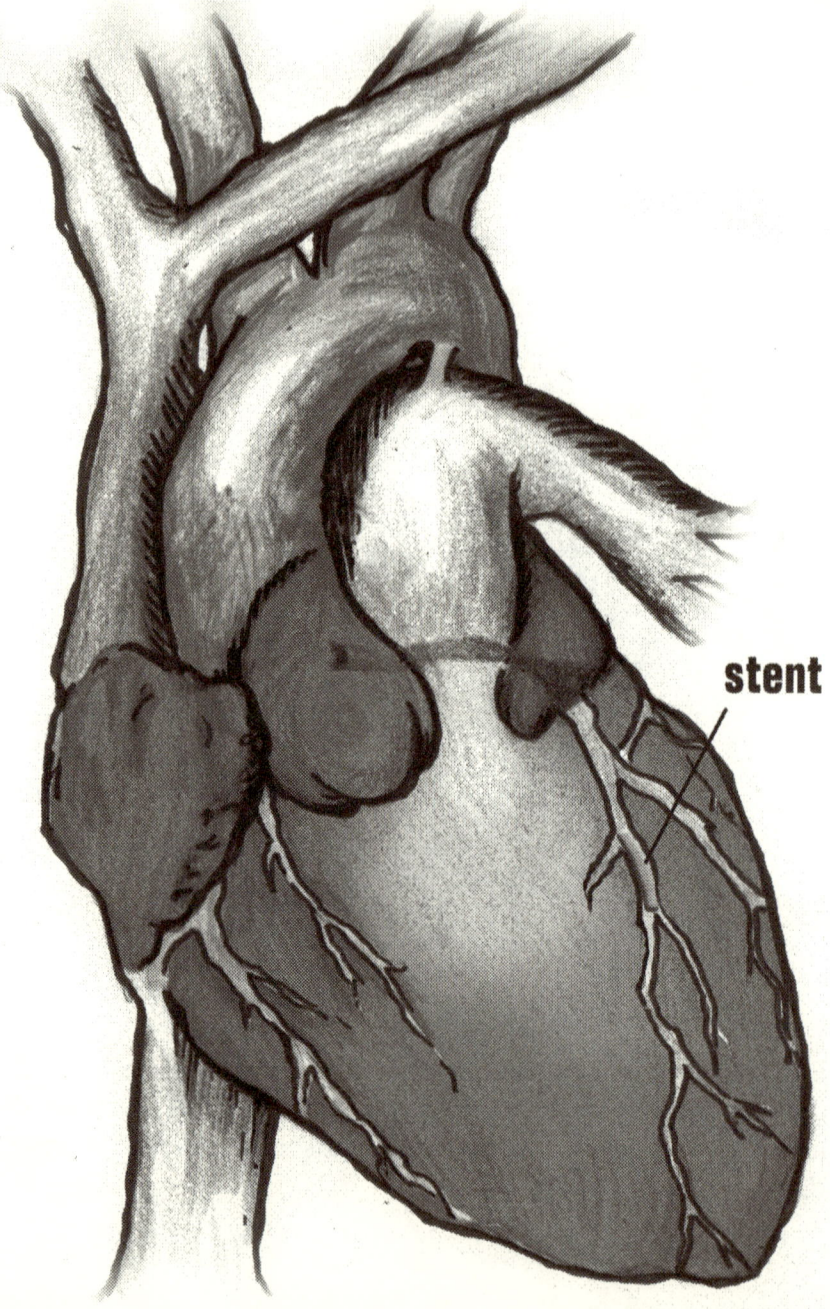

stent

Fig. 2-b. Coronary artery with stent in place, in a previously occluded artery. The stent will hold the artery open (after the angioplasty).

Risk Factor Modification:

What this really means is to try and reduce your possible risks for getting a heart attack. We know that there are certain factors in life that cause early blockages in the coronary arteries. By removing these so-called "risk factors" from your daily life, you can lower the risk that you will get a heart attack, or reduce the possibility of a repeat heart attack. The first risk factor modification that we recommend is to not smoke. In most young people who get heart attacks, such as our Mr. Harrison, we usually find that they were smokers. We frequently observed that they started smoking at a young age. Nicotine raises your blood pressure because it causes your body to release adrenaline, which is a hormone. This hormone makes your blood vessels constrict and your heart beat faster. The nicotine in the bloodstream also inhibits an enzyme, lipoprotein lipase. This is an enzyme, which causes the break down of the bad type of cholesterol, LDL. By smoking, you cause the LDL (bad cholesterol) to be elevated. By stopping smoking, you reduce your risk factor of coronary heart disease. After 2-3 years of not smoking, your risk of coronary artery disease may be as low as a person who never smoked.

What else can you do to lower your risk factors for having a heart attack? Well, the other most important thing is lowering your LDL cholesterol level. We know that the LDL cholesterol causes plaque to build up in your coronary arteries (fig. 2-c). The LDL is the bad cholesterol that gets deposited in the coronary arteries and causes the blockages. By lowering your LDL cholesterol level you can help keep plaque from building up in your arteries. Eating a healthy, low fat diet is a good way to start. If you already have coronary artery disease, your doctor probably wants you to lower your LDL level by at least 30-35% through diet, exercise, and possibly medications. The medications that we most recommend for lowering LDL are the 'statins' such as Crestor, Lipitor, Zocor, or Pravachol, etc.

Sometimes, we find that the person has normal cholesterol and a normal LDL level. However, their HDL cholesterol, i.e., the good cholesterol, may be low. The HDL cholesterol is the type of cholesterol that removes the cholesterol from the coronary arteries so that it may be metabolized in the liver. If you could increase your HDL level to at least 50 you are on the right track. However, there are not a lot of great medications that will raise the HDL level. We know that female hormones raise the HDL level and that is why women are at less risk for a heart attack, than men, at least until they reach menopause. The female hormones drop down to a level comparable to that of a man after menopause. There are certain medications that will raise the HDL, such as Niacin and Tricor. We frequently will use these medications to help increase a patient's serum

HDL. We know that exercise, especially intense aerobic exercise, will also elevate the HDL. Some statins claim to elevate the HDL level, but they work primarily by reducing the LDL cholesterol.

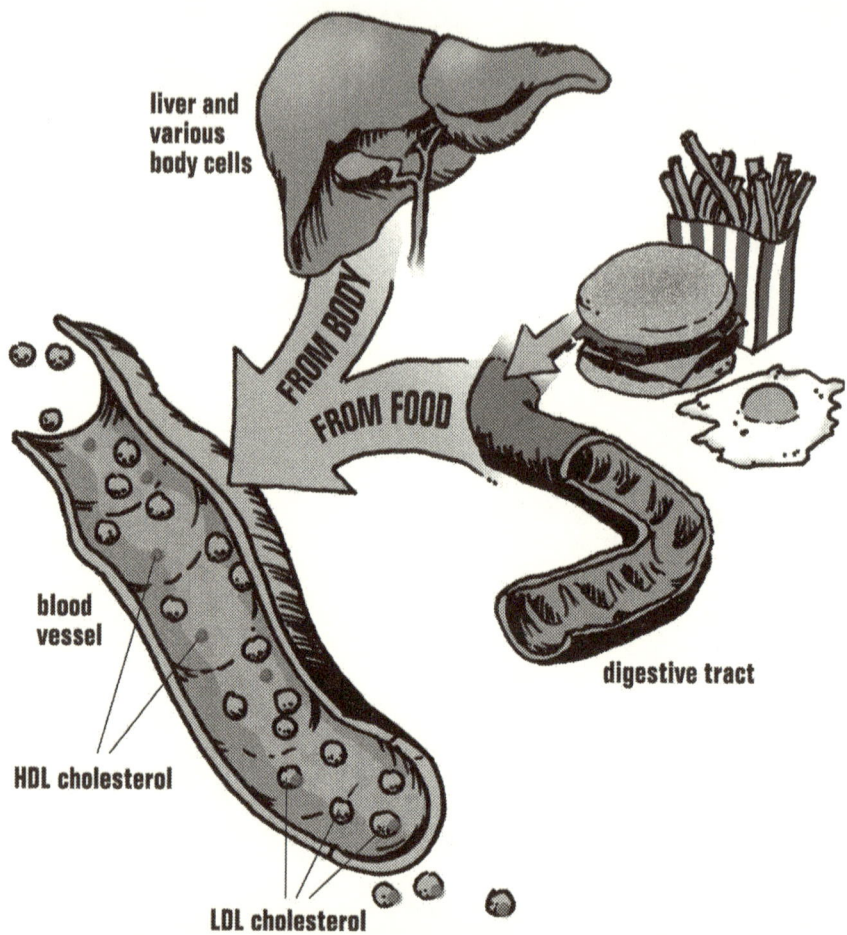

Fig. 2-c. The **LDL-cholesterol**, from food and the liver, gets deposited in the arteries. This is the bad cholesterol.

The **HDL-cholesterol** carries the cholesterol away from the arteries. This is the good cholesterol and you want to have a high HDL-cholesterol.

Other factors that you can do to reduce your risk factors for coronary artery disease is to exercise regularly. Regular exercise can make your heart stronger and reduce your risk of heart disease. I recommend intense aerobic exercise at least four times per week for thirty minutes each time. I personally try to exercise every day for at least one hour, and that is intense aerobic exercise. That does not include my walking, which I do at least 3-4 times per day, as well. (see photo of me with dogs, figure 2-D).

Controlling the blood pressure is another factor, which will lower your risk for heart disease. If you are taking medicine for high blood pressure, be sure that your physician monitors you. Other medications such as aspirin and vitamin E may lower a person's risk of having a heart attack.

Mr. Harrison, after his angioplasty, was put on one aspirin per day and a Beta- blocker. Beta-blockers are medications that have been shown to improve survival in patients who have sustained a myocardial infarction (heart attack).

Beta-blockers will slow the heart rate and lower blood pressure. Mr. Harrison was also placed on Plavix, which is another type of blood thinner, which helps prevent arteries from re-clogging. It also prevents the stent from becoming occluded. He was placed on medicine to help him stop smoking. He was given a Nicotine patch, to reduce the withdrawal from tobacco. That would help reduce his cravings for nicotine and allow him to stop smoking in a sensible manner.

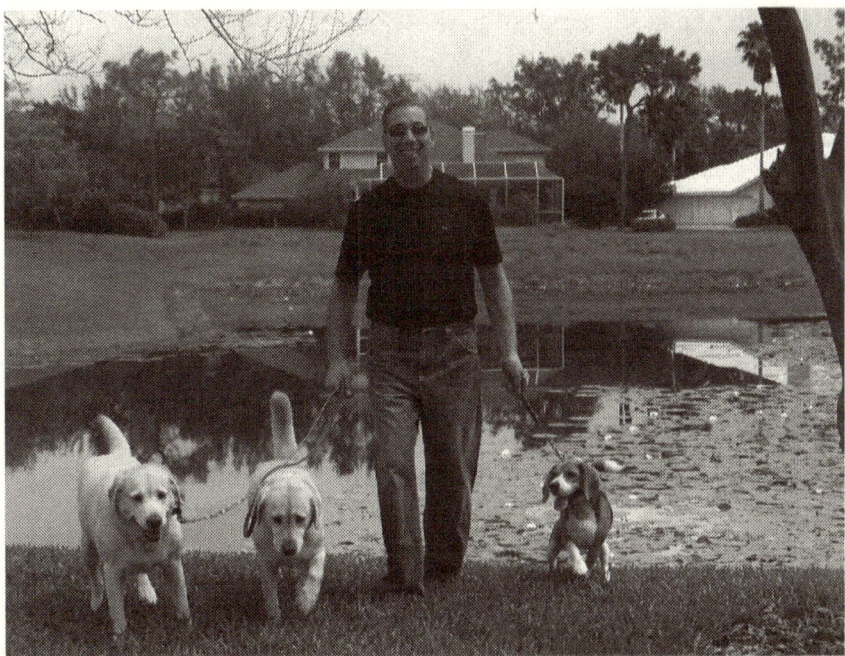

Fig. 2-d. Photo of me with my dogs - exercising. I try to walk with my dogs at least 4 times everyday. That gives us a nice 4 -5 miles per day of relaxed walking. It is good thinking time. I also try to do one hour of aerobic exercise daily - either running, biking, or swimming. This will keep your muscles in tone and the weight down. Exercise is known to raise the HDL-cholesterol and help fight heart disease. Aerobic exercise also has many other benefits - improves your immune system, fights cancer, prevents osteoporosis, and others. In addition, it feels good and can make you happier.

Other risk factors, such as genetics, we are not able to control. Obviously, he could not select his parents and his genes. However, we are able to modify his diet and convince him to stop smoking. He takes aspirin and Plavix as blood thinners, and blood pressure medicine. He has a sensible diet. He has a regular exercise program. Utilizing these measures, Mr. Harrison should do well. Certainly these lifestyle modifications will reduce his risk factors for heart disease. I am concerned that he will not stop smoking and this will need to be monitored.

Special Topic- Acute Coronary Artery Occlusion

Coronary artery disease is the most common type of heart disease affecting over 7 million Americans. It results from atherosclerosis - the gradual build up of plaque from blood vessels that feed your heart (fig. 2-e). Over time, these plaques, which are deposits of fat, cholesterol, calcium, and other cellular sludge from your blood, can narrow your coronary arteries. This could cause less blood flow to the heart muscle and thus less oxygen to the heart muscle tissue. When you get a decreased blood flow to the heart, you could get chest pain, or angina. This is a gradual process and occurs very slowly, over the years.

Just what causes the sudden heart attack? Why does someone go from just a blockage in a coronary artery to all of a sudden having a heart attack? The heart attack is usually due to an acute coronary artery occlusion. This means that one of the arteries leading to the heart muscle suddenly becomes completely blocked. The blockage is not usually due to the plaque itself, but is due to a rupture of a plaque. That means that a part of a plaque will break off and the body tries to repair that plaque (fig. 2-f). It does this by forming a blood clot in the artery, which had been previously partially blocked by plaque. By repairing a ruptured plaque, the whole artery can become occluded by a clot. This is what happens when a patient has a heart attack. This is the reason we give patients aspirin and other blood thinners. The aspirin does nothing to slow the advent of atherosclerosis, in the coronary arteries. What it does is prevent the plaque from filling in with blood clots, and thus occluding the whole artery. Aspirin may prevent an acute heart attack.

What could cause the plaque to rupture? Intense stress can cause epinephrine release. This may result in a tear in the artery that has the large amount of plaque.

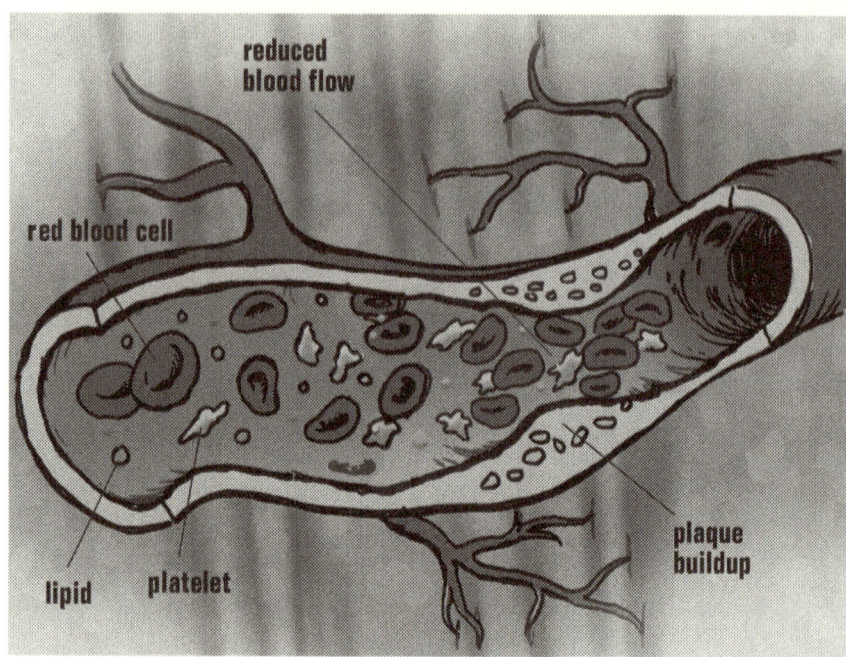

Fig. 2-e. Partially occluded coronary artery with a large amount of plaque on the arterial wall. This **partially** occludes the blood flow through the artery.

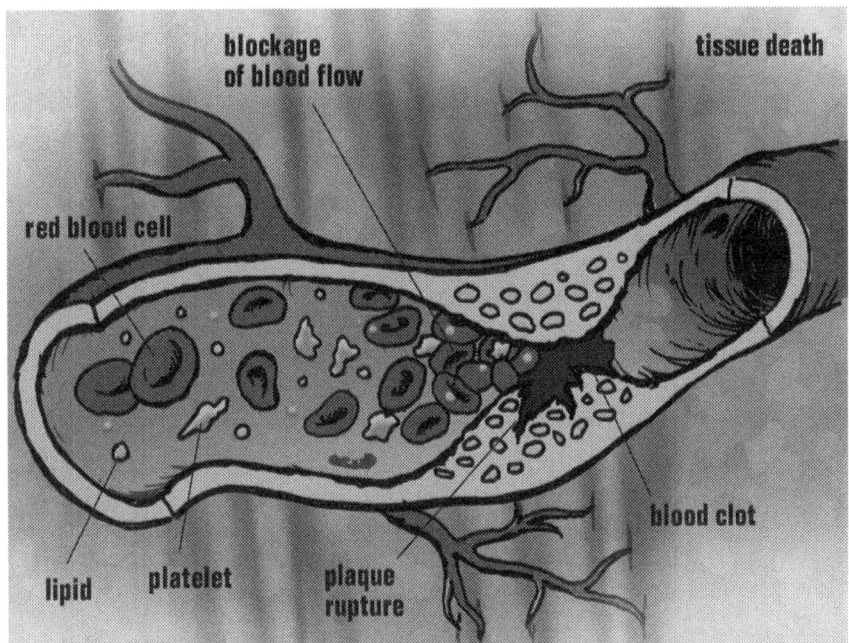

Fig. 2-f. An artery that has a small plaque can become totally occluded rapidly. This happens when the plaque gets a break in it and a clot will form. This clot will **completely** occlude the whole artery.

It is worthwhile noting at this point, that the best prevention against a plaque rupture is not having the plaque develop in the first place. If the plaque does rupture, it is best to be on aspirin and/or Plavix so that the clot will not form and completely occlude the blood vessel.

Truth and Reality

Every patient should do all that is possible to minimize his or her risk of having a heart attack. The same risk factors for a heart attack also apply to a stroke. By reducing your risk factors, one may certainly minimize the possibility of having a heart attack (or a stroke). If you have a strong family predisposition to having heart disease, then you should be evaluated to determine your potential risk for coronary artery disease. Things that should be checked are your blood pressure, smoking history, family genetics, LDL, HDL, and even get a VAP test. This last test will give you more information regarding your types of HDL and LDL that are floating around in your bloodstream. This can tell you if you are at even higher risk than you may think. If you have high blood pressure, this should be aggressively treated to bring it down to approximately 120/80 or even less. Recent studies have shown that lower blood pressure will reduce your risk factors for heart disease or a stroke.

I strongly recommend that if you have two or more risk factors, you get a stress test. If the stress test is in any way inconclusive or suspicious, then you should then undergo a Thallium stress test, i.e., and nuclear stress test. If this is again inconclusive or suspicious and you have a high amount of risk factors, then you should proceed with a cardiac catheterization, to evaluate the coronary arteries. Unfortunately, this is somewhat of an invasive and expensive test. I am hoping that in the near future there will be certain types of scans, which will be noninvasive such as a PET scan or a new CT Scan of the heart. With the new CT or PET scans, the coronary arteries will be able to be visualized without any dyes or needles. You would simply go in for a scan and the doctors would look at your coronary arteries and then determine if you should go for a heart catheterization or not.

If you have high blood pressure, you should be on a very strict diet and exercise program. You should be on medication. If your LDL is elevated or your HDL is suppressed, then you should be on certain medications, as well. In addition, there are some other tests, which can assist in determining your risk for coronary artery disease, such as a C-reactive protein (CRP) and homocysteine levels. However, I do not find these last two tests to contribute to the evaluation of someone for heart disease.

If you have several risk factors or have had a previous heart attack or an angioplasty and a stent placed, you should be on aspirin at 81 milligrams per day. In addition, you should be placed on Plavix at 75 milligrams per day. You should be on these medications unless you have certain conditions that would preclude you from taking them, such as a bleeding disorder or a recent bleeding ulcer, or other problem that would cause you to bleed.

As regards our patient, Mr. Harrison, he certainly helped his disease to progress, by neglecting his health. If he did not smoke, and he had watched his lipid profile, he certainly could have prevented a heart attack from occurring, at such a young age. Once you get a heart attack, some degree of heart muscle tissue is damaged and this may cause a decreased patient survival time.

It is very important for the patient to reduce their risk factors for heart disease, and to take all measures possible to prevent the coronary arteries from becoming occluded. By getting proper medical care and using the proper prevention techniques as outlined above, I believe that a heart attack can be prevented or at least delayed. If coronary artery disease can be identified early, then intensive measures can be implemented by the Physician to prevent further progression of plaque. This will prevent occlusion of the blood vessels and a heart attack.

Summary

Coronary **heart** disease is also called coronary **artery** disease. This occurs when fatty substances called plaques block the coronary arteries. Plaques build up in coronary arteries over years. As plaques get bigger in the coronary arteries, they could reduce blood flow to the heart muscle and thus deprive the heart tissue of oxygen. When the vessel becomes completely occluded, a heart attack can occur.

Plaques are mainly composed of cholesterol. Cholesterol is present in all of our bodies. It is also present in meat and dairy foods. There are several different types of cholesterol including low-density lipoproteins (LDL), which is the bad type of cholesterol, and high-density lipoproteins (HDL), which is the good type of cholesterol. The good cholesterol protects arteries from plaque build up.

There are several ways in which you can prevent your coronary arteries from being blocked by plaque. As in our patient, Mr. Harrison, the number one factor that causes premature, blockage of the coronary arteries is smoking cigarettes. Nicotine raises your blood pressure and makes your blood vessels constrict and your heart beat faster. It also prevents a break down of certain fats in the blood and causes premature atherosclerosis of the coronary arteries.

Genetics is another important factor in promoting heart disease, in patients that are predisposed to coronary artery disease. If your parents or aunts and uncles or grandparents had heart disease at a young age, then you will be much more inclined to do so as well. It is very important to select your parents and have good genes. Unfortunately, that is out of our control. So, the things that we can do, is to control some of the risk factors, which are preventable. We need to keep our cholesterol as low as possible, especially the LDL cholesterol. The recent literature has demonstrated that an LDL below 70 is the objective. This is especially true if you have any risk factors for Coronary Artery DISEASE. This can be done through diet, exercise, and medications. If your cholesterol is high and you have a family predisposition towards coronary artery disease, I suggest you get on a lipid-lowering agent. The medicine that I prescribe the most, which I find to be the most effective at this point, is <u>Crestor</u>. This is in the class of medications called "statins". They work by lowering the cholesterol at the level of the liver. You need to have your liver tests checked every 3 months for a year. Crestor also can raise the HDL (the good cholesterol). Other medicines in this class that are also very effective are Lipitor, Zocor, Pravachol, and Lescol. Crestor is the medicine that is marketed as having the least amount of side effects, in this class of medications.

Controlling your blood pressure is also important. High blood pressure (hypertension) can cause a plaque to rupture and could cause an acute coronary artery occlusion - a sudden heart attack. There are many ways in which blood pressure can be reduced, but the most common is with medication. If you have coronary artery disease and hypertension, medication is especially important. I would suggest an ACE inhibitor (ACEI), or angiotensin-converting enzyme inhibitor, such as Altace. You can also use an angiotensin receptor blocker (ARB) such as Benicar. Other medications, which are extremely effective, are beta- blockers such as Tenormin, Toprol, or Lopressor, and calcium channel blockers such as Norvasc or Cardizem. Exercise is another method, which can make your heart stronger and reduce your risk of heart disease. Exercise can also help reduce your cholesterol and your blood pressure. I suggest intense aerobic exercise at least 4-6 times per week.

A low dose of aspirin such as 81 milligrams per day of a coated aspirin can help prevent an acute coronary occlusion. This has some risks, especially bleeding problems. One may also consider Plavix as an anticoagulant, either in addition to or instead of Aspirin. The combination of Aspirin and Plavix is essential for anyone that has had a stent placed. There is an increased risk of bleeding with this combination of medicines. You should discuss this with your physician.

Vitamin supplements such as vitamin E may lower a person's risk of having a heart attack. People at risk of a heart attack or stroke may also wish to take antioxidants. However, recent studies have **not** shown that the vitamins really have any beneficial effect in reducing the risk for coronary artery disease.

The evaluation and treatment for coronary artery disease are changing rapidly. With new non-invasive scans, we may be able to visualize the coronary arteries without any dye being injected. The new stents and drugs for opening the arteries are evolving rapidly. This is a field of medicine that is progressing very fast and is extremely exciting to watch.

3 | Obesity, Diabetes, and Weight Loss

"You don't have to cook fancy or complicated masterpieces - just good food from fresh ingredients."

Julia Child (1912 - 2004)

It was a rainy Tuesday morning in the clinic. I was seeing one patient after the other. The clinic gets quite busy in the mornings. Most people always seem to be in a hurry. Everyone wants to be seen with a minimum of waiting time. There were the usual follow-up patients to examine and talk with. There were patients with heart disease and diabetes and other medical problems. Since I have many years of experience, I was able to make important medical decisions, on a rapid basis. I was able to change medications, order tests, and examine patients, without much difficulty. Even though I was seeing a lot of patients, and many of them were quite ill, I was able to handle the problems easily. It was basically a standard morning for me. It was kind of like long-distance running - you get in the zone and time just goes by. However, you never know what type of emergency will come in next, and break up the easy, early morning routine.

The rooms were wet from the rain and there was a musty smell in the air. Some patients were sicker than others and required more attention. Others just needed to be reassured that everything was okay. I was evaluating a patient with heart disease. He just had a heart bypass and was looking better than before the surgery. His scar down his chest was healing and he was able to breathe without a pillow on his chest. That was a major accomplishment for him. I was talking to him about his diet and medications, when a nurse came into the room without knocking. That was unusual of Jane, and cause for concern. Jane was an experienced nurse and didn't get rattled unless there was a major problem. She said, "There's a hot one in room 10 - better come quickly."

I scurried over to the other examining room. We didn't talk in the hallways and I didn't know what was going on with the next patient. This was the moment of truth in medicine. There really was no excitement like it in the world. Someone is very ill and possibly dying just feet away from you. They needed me to get there quickly. I knew that I had the knowledge and skills to save somebody. Everyone was depending on me. This is a co-dependent's dream. I became focused and entered the exam room.

Being a doctor and taking care of an acutely ill patient is different than power. It is the accumulation of years of training and clinical skills. It is the feeling that you can actually help and make a difference in someone's life. As we approached the room, there was already a flurry of activity going on. I saw the EKG tech running into the room. Someone else was bringing an oxygen canister and other supplies into the exam room. The crash cart was already opened and the seal was broken. All of these were signs that we need to work quickly and efficiently. You needed to have grace under pressure. Never panic and always stay calm. That is what I always told myself.

My first glance at the patient told me that this was serious. It was a young lady. She was huffing and puffing for air. Every breath was rapid and short. She was straining to breath and her color was not good. I looked at the EKG and her heart rate was about 160 beats per minute. Her beautiful chestnut brown hair was matted to her scalp. She was sweating profusely. The patient was restless and was trying to be calmed down by the nurses. She was very agitated and could not be calmed down. I spotted her husband in the corner with a sad, pathetic look on his face. He was pleading for help with his eyes, and his own helplessness showed in his expression. There was a new odor in the air - a fruity smell, like that of an old packet of gum. It was a sweet smell, but distinctly unpleasant. I thought

I knew immediately what was going on and what needed to be done.

The patient was Lisa Thornton. I knew her for several years. She was a very sweet young lady and had recently married, and had a baby. She had a difficult pregnancy due to gestational diabetes. Her blood sugar had gone up during the pregnancy. This was not very uncommon. While she was pregnant, she monitored her sugars very closely and took insulin as needed. We sent her to a high-risk Obstetrician and I lost track of her after that. During her pregnancy, she put on over 100 pounds and her diabetes went out of control. The nurse took her accucheck (blood sugar level) in the office. Her sugar was 453 (normal 80-125). She was in diabetic ketoacidosis and was very ill.

Lisa stopped taking her insulin after the delivery of her baby. She later told me that she became depressed and gave up on watching her diet. She stopped taking her medications. With her post-partum depression in full swing, she started eating everything in sight. She and her husband frequented the local buffet restaurants, loading their plates with as much food as possible. She now weighed 325 pounds. I hardly recognized her. She had stopped caring about her personal appearance due to the post-partum depression. Her husband didn't know what to do either. They stopped communicating with each other and dropped out of the medical community. She was very depressed after her delivery and stopped going to the doctors. This was a dangerous situation.

We treated her rapidly in the office, giving her large quantities of intravenous (IV) fluids. We also gave her an injection of insulin to bring down her blood sugar. She was fortunate that we had the supplies and equipment to take care of her problem. In addition, Lisa was lucky that we were able to recognize her problem and take care of it right away. Ms. Thornton was brought to the hospital by ambulance. She was actually looking better as she was being taken out of the office on a stretcher. Her breathing and pulse had quieted down and she regained some of the color in her face.

I went to see her in the hospital later that day. She was doing much better and was able to talk with me. It always amazed me how people with this condition will get better so rapidly. Diabetes out of control (Diabetic ketoacidosis) is treated with a combination of fluids and insulin. They usually perk right up. After a few days in the hospital, she did really well. It was lucky that she was so young; otherwise she may not have fared so well. The body tries to get rid of the sugar (glucose) in the bloodstream by making you urinate a lot. This makes the patient very dehydrated and acidotic. The treatment is easy and the patient can get better quite quickly. However, they need to get proper treatment quickly, or the situation can be fatal. If a patient is older, the stress of diabetic ketoacidosis on the body can be lethal.

Lisa developed diabetes in her late twenties during pregnancy. All of her family members are diabetic, and developed the disease at the same age. That is, they developed Type II diabetes due to obesity and overeating. They all had put on tens of pounds and became obese. Their bodies would develop an **insulin resistance** and diabetes would come on like a "horse out of the gate". When a person becomes overweight, the body develops a resistance to insulin, which is a hormone that helps to process sugars. Due to the resistance of the body against the effects of insulin, the body undergoes many changes. The pancreas that produces insulin secretes more insulin into the bloodstream. Patients that are overweight or obese, have high amounts of insulin floating in their bloodstream. The insulin is also a "storage hormone". It works by making sugar go into cells and converting other sugars into fats. The fats then get stored in different areas of the body. In men, the fat gets stored in the lower abdomen. In women, the fat is stored in the thighs and buttocks. The fatter one gets, the more that resistance will develop. This means that when you eat, the body will produce more insulin. This is to overcome the resistance of the body to the insulin. When you have a high insulin level, any food that you eat will be rapidly converted to fat and stored in the body. Obesity will almost guarantee that you will be even fatter due to the insulin resistance. It is a **cycle** that is self-perpetuating and can cause many problems for so many people.

So, what happened to Lisa? She put on a massive amount of weight in a short period of time, during her pregnancy. While she was pregnant, she was getting good medical care. She was on insulin and her blood sugars were being monitored. After her pregnancy, she continued to eat excessively. She became depressed and stopped monitoring her sugars and taking her insulin. As she put on more weight, the body attempted to control her blood sugars by producing more insulin. She stopped taking her medications, and this exacerbated her medical problems. Her blood sugars then became so high and the body wasn't able to process them effectively. This led to an acidosis and her becomingly seriously ill.

Her problem was not directly from the diabetes. She only developed the diabetes as a consequence of being extremely overweight. This was also true of the other members of her family. They all had an insulin resistance that led to increased amounts of insulin being produced. This caused more fat deposition and further insulin resistance and even more weight gain. They all continued to spiral downward to further weight gain and worsening diabetes.

How come not all obese people are diabetics? This is due to certain people being able to process their blood glucose. However, most obese people will still have very high insulin levels and insulin resistance. This will still cause sugars to be converted to fat and stored in our bodies, in places that we don't want them. I treat so many patients for diabetes as well as other problems secondary to obesity. Many obese patients have high blood pressure, heart disease, strokes, bad arthritis, low back pain, as well as a host of other ailments related to being overweight. As doctors, we usually treat the problem and not the underlying cause. For example, if a person who is severely overweight (a BMI of over 35) develops high blood pressure, they will get a pill to bring down the blood pressure. However, the underlying problem is usually the obesity. The obesity is what should be treated, in addition to the high blood pressure. Frequently, a patient that loses weight from dieting will no longer require medications for high blood pressure or diabetes.

After Lisa became better from the diabetes attack, we spoke a lot. She told me that she started putting on weight when she became pregnant. Her husband would make fun of her and call her names. He would ridicule her for being heavy. This made her more depressed and she would even eat more. She felt that she would lose the weight after she had the baby. She had a difficult pregnancy and couldn't exercise. Lisa was placed on bed-rest for most of the pregnancy. She also said that it was too hard to make the foods that were healthy for her. Her husband wanted certain foods and they ate a lot of sweets. She stated, "I usually ate what he did to make him feel good". She didn't want him to feel bad about his eating high calorie foods. She would join him in eating large quantities of high calorie foods. They would often go to the restaurants that had buffets, and eat as much as possible. They "always got their money's worth".

As she became heavier, her depression became worse. Her clothes stopped fitting right. Lisa knew that she had to stop eating so much, but the food was like a drug - she couldn't stop the madness. She would eat when she felt sad. Nobody could control her eating and certainly she ate even when she wasn't hungry. She told me that she tried to go to a Weight Watchers meeting. Going to one of the meetings, made her so depressed that she never went back. She counted the points and would lie to herself about how many points she had consumed. "We won't count this candy bar, since it is a reward for walking today".

She stopped drinking diet sodas. She would stop at a convenience store and get the large drinks. These contain high amounts of high-fructose corn syrup (HFCS). This compound is cheaper than sugar. It also causes an intense release of insulin. This is one of the main culprits in making America fat - avoid sodas and foods with HFCS!

About a week after her hospital discharge from the diabetes attack, Lisa came to my office. She looked a lot better and was very kind, but so vulnerable. She had a hard time talking about her weight gain. Her obesity caused her to be so embarrassed. She weighed 315 pounds. We talked about the different options to lose the weight. There was no easy fix. The main problem was to keep the diabetes under control and prevent another episode of acidosis. I adjusted her medications and suggested that she get marriage counseling. She was under a lot of pressure to keep her husband happy, and felt that she was the cause of the problems in the marriage. "If only I could get thin, then our marriage would be great". We talked about the different options that were available for her. There are a host of pills that can curb the appetite - Meridia, Adipex, Fastin, and others. These all work by suppressing the appetite in the brain. They also cause the stomach to constrict and make people feel full. However, there are so many side effects, such as high blood pressure, cardiac arrhythmias, valve problems, (remember Phen-fen). There is Xenical that blocks the body's ability to absorb fat. However, this can cause oily diarrhea and is extremely unpleasant. There is a **gastric bypass surgery**. To my surprise, she wanted to try diet and exercise as her option for weight loss. She was on an antidepressant and I think this curbed her appetite. Several months later, she had lost over 100 pounds and felt and looked much healthier. She started to work out on a regular basis and stopped eating anything not on her prescribed diet plan.

Lisa didn't need to take insulin injections anymore. She was able to take pills for her diabetes and this was kept under good control. We had previously referred her to a Psychiatrist and he placed her on anti-depressants. Her post-partum depression had resolved and she started to enjoy her life. Lisa had to work hard at losing the weight, but she did it and had great resolve to become healthy again.

4 | Treatment of Obesity and Weight Loss

"Can't Anyone Tell Me How to Lose This Weight?"
(lament of most people trying to lose weight)

Rosemary Coleman is a patient that I had known for many years. One day she had come into the office, not looking like her usual self. She was a beautiful, young woman, about 35 years old. (My definition of young has recently changed; thirty-five is definitely a lot younger than it used to be.) Anyway, she was tall and skinny. At least she had been skinny for the last ten years. Her workouts had been exhausting and she always managed to stay in shape. She had been meticulous in her appearance. Her hair, when I had seen her at her previous visit, was shiny and full and always coiffed perfectly. She was solely responsible for the depletion of the ozone with all of her hair spray usage. Now she appeared different. Her appearance had definitely deteriorated. Ever since she had lost weight, following her gastric bypass, about ten years ago, she always wore tight clothes. She said that she always felt like

Professor Crump in the Nutty Professor "Spandex, I want to wear Spandex."

Rosemary had lost over 150 pounds since her gastric bypass. This was just a little more that ten years ago. She subsequently had to undergo several plastic surgery procedures to tighten her skin and remove some skin folds. However, she had done very well. She had felt great and gained confidence in herself. She loved being skinny and thought that this was the best thing that happened to her. Food no longer had its hold on her and she was free from its clutches. Rosemary was fat from childhood. People made fun of her as early as she was able to remember. She didn't know why she overate, but she did eat nonetheless. As a pre-teen, her peers frequently ridiculed her. Boys would never ask her out and she became very shy and introverted. She would promise herself that she would never eat again and would then eat twice as much. Rosemary was very unhappy and thought of suicide many times as a young woman. Nobody asked her to her high school prom and she did not go. She didn't want to be seen alone and not having fun as did everybody else. Sports were not for her either. She was not able to participate on any of the school teams popping up for girls and young women. Cheerleading and dance squads were also out of the question. Her weight in high school was over 325 pounds. This made her so unhappy and she didn't know what to do. She tried all of the diet and everything was unsuccessful. Diet pills only made her edgy and she ate even when she wasn't hungry and had no appetite.

She loved to read and was a voracious consumer of books. Love stories were her favorite and she dreamed of one day falling in love. But, how could anyone possibly love her. She suffered from a low self-esteem, and felt that no one could possible care for her. She went to college and became an over-achiever. She excelled in every subject and her professors thought that she was brilliant. However, she was deeply troubled and very unhappy. Then, one day, she heard about the gastric bypass surgery. She thought that would be the answer to her problems. That would be perfect for her. In fact, she was the ideal candidate for the procedure. In 1995, at the age of twenty-five, she underwent a gastric bypass procedure. This worked perfectly for her. She had a massive and rapid weight loss. For the first time in her life, she was thin. Of course, there were side effects. She developed nausea and vomiting for months after the procedure. She had to undergo some plastic surgeries on her abdomen and arms to remove loose skin. However, these were minor compared to the joy she felt in being thin. She now felt " normal."

I last saw her about six months ago. She looked very different now. She appeared too thin. Her hair was no longer lustrous, but sparse and straw-like. Her skin was gaunt and had a grayish shade. Her eyes were pale and sunken. When she walked, she became short of breath and easily fatigued. Rosemary told me that she had been having some stomach discomfort. Her appetite was less than ever and she couldn't even force herself to eat. She told me "I am living on juices and Tums and over-the-counter Prilosec. I feel terrible. I have pins and needles in my arms and legs. My skin is always tingling. I haven't even been able to take my vitamins. When I start to eat I get so nauseous and I immediately have to stop eating. I eat mainly ice chips. I am happy that I am thin, but I am too sick to enjoy it. I could hardly walk." My response was deliberate and thoughtful "let's take a look and see what's going on."

I asked her to disrobe and get on the examining table. We talked while I did my exam. She was in a patient gown and she talked while I listened to her heart and lungs. She told me that she had tried every diet that was known, prior to her gastric bypass. She really didn't want the surgery, but she felt that she had no alternative. She was apologizing for having undergone the gastric bypass. Rosemary felt guilty that she was now sick and this was due to the gastric bypass. She didn't understand why she was ill and couldn't eat anything.

A gastric bypass (fig. 4-a, b) is certainly an interesting phenomenon that is sweeping America and Europe. It is definitely an extreme measure to take to lose weight. People who elect to have gastric bypass surgery are at least 100 pounds overweight. This is an alternative to dieting and should be considered in patients with certain health problems who need rapid weight loss. The actual surgery **alters your digestive system** by closing off parts of your stomach to make it smaller. This then restricts the amount of food your stomach can hold and the amount of food that you can eat. Some versions of the surgery can make a bypass of the small intestine. In other words, a direct connection is made between your stomach and small intestine.

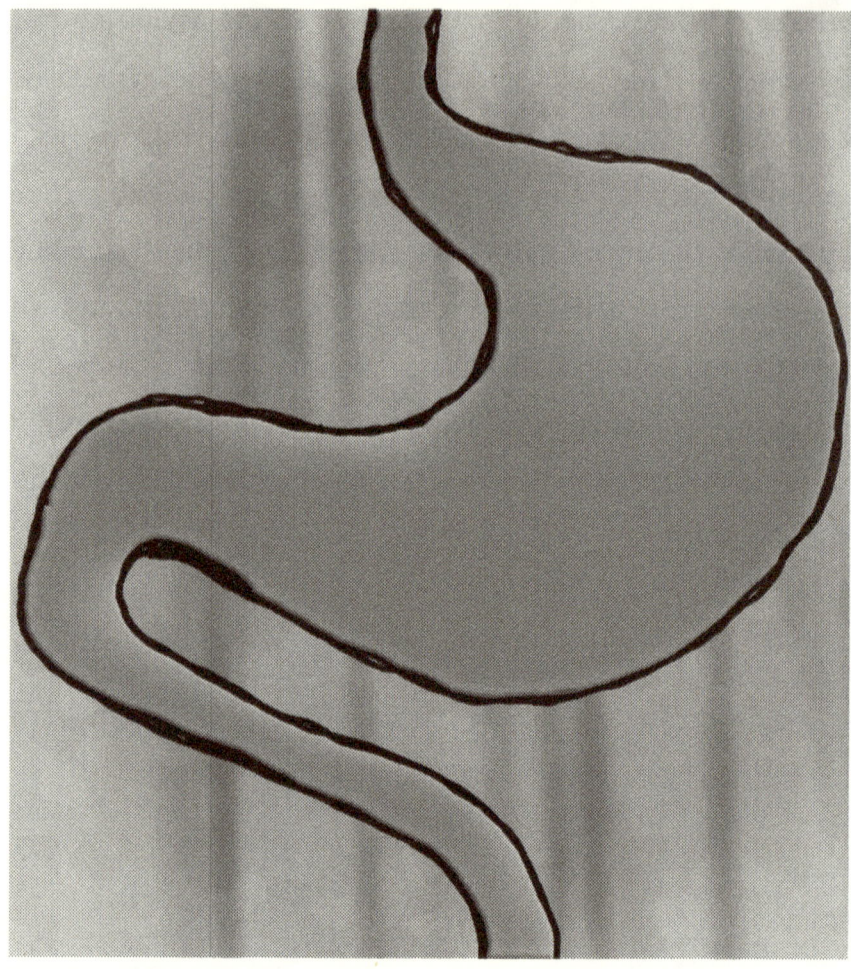

Fig. 4-a. Picture of a normal stomach and intestines.

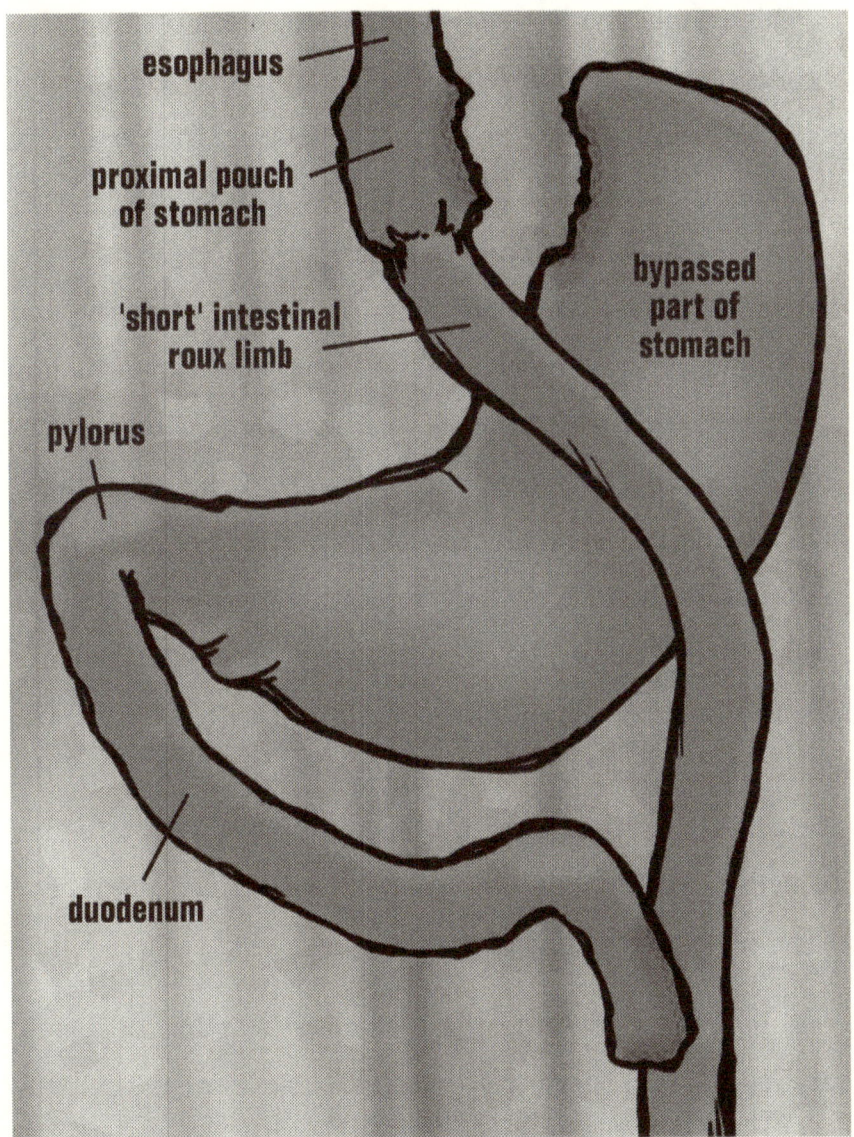

Fig. 4-b. Picture of a stomach and intestines **after a gastric bypass.**

This connection bypass is part of the digestive tract that absorbs calories and nutrients. This certainly can lead to some major side effects and complications. Despite the possibility of multiple side effects, this procedure is becoming a very common type of surgery. I have had multiple patients in my practice who have had this type of bariatric surgery, and many have done extremely well. I have others who are having side effects, such as lots of nausea, vomiting, kidney stones and infections. The gastric bypass surgery is not to be taken casually and it is generally recommended for people that are over double their ideal body weight and have failed other types of weight loss. The surgery has both risks and benefits so careful discussion with the surgeon is very important. The aim of the surgery is to reduce the amount of food that the stomach can hold so that people feel full if they eat more than a small meal. People who exceed the prescribed amount of eating usually feel uncomfortable or even sick.

Other types of surgery are stomach stapling or gastric banding. This surgery creates a small pouch at the top of the stomach. The pouch is not completely closed off from the rest of the stomach. There is a small opening that allows some food to pass into the stomach and then into the intestines. This stapling or banding is done so that the stomach gets small enough so that you can only eat a small amount of food, approximately one cup of food before feeling uncomfortable.

Approximately 80 percent of people who undergo stomach stapling, banding or bypass will achieve weight loss. One-third of all people having surgery for obesity develop gallstones or nutritional deficiency, such as anemia and osteoporosis. There will be a new type of procedure that will be very popular in the United States. This is the gastric stimulator. This consists of two wires that are placed around the sides of the stomach and operated through a little battery-pack, located under the skin. This will activate and squeeze the stomach shut so you will have the sensation of being full. This is much less traumatic than having bypass surgery on the stomach or a banding procedure. I do believe that within the next year or two this will be the most common type of bariatric surgery to be performed, as the side effects will be minimal, or at least a lot less than a full gastric bypass surgical procedure.

So what happened to our lovely Rosemary? Why did she get so sick, many years after her procedure? Well, she developed a Vitamin B-12 deficiency. This vitamin is absorbed only in people with an intact stomach. She stopped taking her Vitamin B-12 injections and became sick. These effects of Vitamin B-12 deficiency are both anemia and neurologic symptoms. She became very weak and fatigued. She was dizzy and had tingling (paresthesias) in her arms and legs. This was the clue to what she had - both anemia and neurologic symptoms. After a few injections of Vitamin B-12, she became much better and her symptoms had resolved. All patients with a gastric bypass should be on monthly injections of Vitamin B-12. I do believe that the gastric bypass was right for Rosemary. However, she did need more careful follow-up and to be reminded never to stop her vitamins. In addition, she was taking antacids and this could prevent further Vitamin B-12 absorption, and she needed to be careful with antacids.

Weight Loss Guidelines:

Truth and Reality:

Calories In - Calories Out = Weight lost or Gained.

This is the basic truth about weight management. If you consume more calories than you expend, then you will gain weight. Conversely, if you take in fewer calories than you burn, then you will lose weight. Unfortunately, there is no easy way to lose weight. One simply has to burn more calories than they can eat. This is the basic premise of weight loss: eat less and burn more calories.

Easier said than done! Weight loss has turned into a multi-billion dollar industry by trying to give people an easy way to lose weight. So many of my patients say that they hardly eat and don't understand why they can't lose weight. The basic fact is that they are still consuming too many calories and not burning off adequate calories to lose weight. In reality, it is almost impossible to lose weight by exercise alone. Unless you are a marathon runner or someone that exercises for hours each day, it is almost impossible to lose weight with exercise alone. **Diet is the mainstay of any weight loss program!**

Here are some diets to follow and help with your weight loss. Remember, no eating in between meals and no drinks with sugar. If you can stay with this program, you will lose weight. I recommend that every person, keep a log of everything that they eat - everything! Do not show this log to anyone but your doctor. Here are some easy diets to follow:

Diet #1

Breakfast: One medium bagel with margarine, coffee with low fat milk and a glass of orange juice. You can substitute tea for the coffee or another low-fat drink. Instead of the bagel, you may have some cereal or a low-fat granola bar. A smoothie can be used instead of fruit for any breakfast or - in-between snack.

Mid-morning snack: Have a fruit of your choice.

Lunch: Chicken pita. Have three ounces of cooked chicken, one whole-wheat pita bread, tomato and a bottle of water.

Snack: Have one-half cup of raw carrots.

Dinner: Have fish, such as halibut, red snapper. One cup of cooked rice a vegetable of choice with assorted seasonings. You may have a slice of bread. Start with a salad with a low fat dressing. If you don't like fish - you can have a chicken breast instead or a turkey burger.

Mid-evening snack: Have a banana or strawberries or yogurt or a low fat ice cream one-quarter cup.

You may also have ices with no sugar and no calories at any time during the day.

Diet # 2

Breakfast: Have an English muffin or a bowl of low fat cereal with skim milk, coffee or tea, banana or strawberries.

Mid-morning: May have a low fat granola bar. If you are going to workout, have a smoothie before - filled with fruit and protein powder.

Lunch: Have a turkey sandwich using low fat turkey, lettuce, tomato, mustard and even a side salad with low fat dressing or vinegar or lemon juice. You can make a fresh turkey and have sandwiches from it all week long.

Mid-afternoon snack: Should be apple, orange or fruit of your choice. A smoothie can be substituted for any snack or breakfast.

Dinner: Have baked chicken, which has been cooked skinless, mashed potatoes and vegetable of your choice.

Evening snack: Should be fresh fruit, a half cup of canned fruit. Remember - ices can be eaten at any time.

Diet #3

Breakfast: Have toast in the morning with margarine, low fat granola bar and a fruit of your choice, as well as a glass of orange juice and caffeine - may be coffee or tea.

Mid-morning snack: Can be fruit of choice, including watermelon, strawberries, grapes, banana, berries, etc.

Lunch: Sandwich of choice, roast beef, turkey, and tuna fish with low fat mayonnaise on toast or rye bread or whole wheat. Use lettuce, tomato, mustard, and avoid mayonnaise.

Dinner: Can be an egg omelet with low fat cheese, cod or flounder, or tofu. You may have a half of a cup of cooked vegetables and a baked potato with margarine or low cholesterol butter.

Evening: May have an 8-ounce, non-fat yogurt or fruit of choice, popcorn, which should be low fat and low sodium.

If you are working out or just get very hungry during the day, you need to eat something. We can't work out if we are drained and have a low blood sugar. I suggest that you get a high power blender for home and work. Make a smoothie or a fruit juice and you can gain energy and feel full. You will also get a lot of fiber and vitamins. Place the following items in a blender until it is liquidy and enjoy. I like to have these types of drinks for breakfast. They are filling, taste great, and don't leave me fatigued after a sugar or caffeine rush - like cake and caffeine does.

Smoothie 1

- 2 cups of ice

- One half apple

- 5 strawberries

-A slice of watermelon or cantaloupe

-Any other fruit that you like

-A squirt of honey

-Protein powder or egg white powder

Smoothie 2

  - 2 cups of ice

  - 1 cup of low-fat milk

  -A sprinkle of low-fat chocolate powder

  -A banana

  - Protein powder

  - Any fruit that you like

Smoothie 3

Take one medium banana, one-half cup of strawberries, 4 ounces of non fat vanilla yogurt, 3 ounces of mixed fruit juice, ice and put it into a blender. You have got a great filling snack and that can be consumed in the morning or evening. You can have half the smoothie before a workout and the rest afterwards.

If you get very hungry during the day, you could certainly pick up an apple, fruit of choice, ices, or popcorn. You can munch on some low fat pretzels but keep the munching and grazing to a minimum. At any time during the day, if you are extremely hungry and just need to have something to fill you up, you can have a smoothie. Take one medium banana, one-half cup or strawberries, 4 ounces of non fat vanilla yogurt, 3 ounces of mixed fruit juice, ice and put it into a blender and you have got a great filling snack and that can be done in the morning or evening. If you are going to do a workout, the smoothie can be an "after-workout treat".

Be very careful of **fad diets.** They may work for a short period of time. They are very difficult to sustain. After a short period of weight loss, the patient will usually rebound and gain more weight. It is better to lose weight sensibly with a good and sustainable program. Some crash diets can actually hurt people by eliminating essential vitamins from their diets. What does work is changing your eating habits and getting on an adequate exercise program. Here are some of the major weight loss plans and their benefits and drawbacks:

These diets in a recent study at Tufts - New England Medical Center in Boston, showed that there is a 42% dropout rate. The differences among the regimens failed to reach statistical significance. In other words, it really didn't matter which diet you were on. The results were similar. There was about a 10-pound weight loss on the people that stayed on the diets.

1. The **Abs Diet** - This is a diet that requires you to be on low carbohydrate, high fiber foods. They suggest that you eat vegetables, low-fat dairy, lean meats, eggs, cereals, and

oatmeal. You should avoid fatty meats and processed foods. This is a lifelong diet and combines diet with workouts to build muscle. In other words, you need to be on a diet and do weight training. This is great for young, athletic people. It works less for older, sedentary types.

2. The **Atkins Diet** - This plan urges you to eat meats and shellfish, eggs, cheese, butter, vegetable oils, and Atkins foods. It restricts fruit, bread, pasta, alcohol, and diary. They suggest daily exercise and are a phased plan. That means that there is a diet for initial weight loss and then one for maintenance.

3. The **DASH Diet** - this diet suggests a high intake of grains and vegetables and fruit. Restricted foods are meat and poultry to very small daily servings and sweets only once a day. This is a lifelong diet program.

4. **Dean Ornish. Program** - this is a low-fat high carbohydrate diet. He suggests that you consume meat, lean poultry, fish, and use vitamins. He advises you to avoid processed and high-fat foods. Also, sugar, caffeine, and alcohol and salt are restricted. This is a lifelong diet and also emphasizes exercise as part of the program.

5. **Jenny Craig Diet Program** - This program uses its proprietary meals and supplements in addition to fruits and

vegetables. You are only allowed to use their proprietary foods and supplements. There is a one-one counseling program and exercise is advised.

6. **Pritikin Eating Plan** - Use of a very low-fat and low-carbohydrate and low-sodium diet. You should have a high daily intake of grains and starches plus green, yellow, orange vegetables, fruits low-fat dairy and low-fat poultry and meat. The use of dairy, eggs, animal fats and oils and salt are restricted. This diet has a lifestyle education plan and regular exercise and is a lifelong program.

7. **South Beach Diet** - use only lean meats, poultry, seafood, fat-free dairy, eggs, low-calorie sweets. This diet works in phases and the second phase allows fruits and whole grains. No fatty meats, dairy, pasta, bread, rice, fruit, or alcohol for the first 14 days. Some fruits are allowed in the second phase, but continued limits on carbohydrates are urged. This diet also suggests daily weight training and vigorous exercise. Go on to the phase 3 for maintenance.

8. **The Ultimate Weight Solution** - This is a high-protein diet. It is recommended that you have 3 proteins, 3 carbohydrates, 4 vegetables, 2 dairies, plus their proprietary foods. Cheeses and other fats are restricted. No " foods you grab on the run" are allowed. This program includes aerobic exercise and is a lifelong commitment.

9. **Weight Watchers Diet Program** - This system focuses on calorie content of food. It works on a point system and the points are based on the fat, fiber, and calories of the food. They suggest increased physical exercise and are a lifelong program.

It really doesn't matter which diet you choose to follow.

If you are committed to weight loss, any of the diets will help you to get some weight off. It is just a matter of not straying from the diet and completing the plan as directed. If you want to make your own foods and enjoy shopping and cooking, avoid the dietary plans with the proprietary foods.

What about **pills**? There is no effortless way to lose weight. We all want a miracle pill or easy program to take our weight off for us. There are millions of gimmicks, tapes, powders, pills, diet programs, etc. The weight-loss industries will rake-in 48 billion in revenues, by the year 2006. There are so many scams and rip-offs out there. People are so desperate to lose weight that they will do anything and pay any amount of money for help. Be especially cautious of the products you see on TV or read in magazines. Most weight loss ads are deceiving and outright false and misleading. I love the one for fat-burners and "Lose weight while you sleep." Of course you lose weight while you sleep - it is the only time you're not eating. In addition, during the night you get a surge of growth hormone that will help you to lose weight. Be very wary of ads that say "Doctor endorsed" or "scientifically -proven to work". That doesn't say which Doctor approved it or was there good scientific studies behind this product.

There is no magic pill for weight loss. In certain cases, if the patient has a Body Mass Index (BMI) over 30, I may prescribe a weight loss pill. This will "jump-start" their weight loss program and help them in the early stages. However, there are many side effects to diet pills. I usually prescribe **Adipex-P**, which is an amphetamine -like medication. This has to be done under strict supervision and close monitoring. The Adipex-P is also known as Phentermine and works by constricting the stomach. The side effects are constipation, irritability, insomnia, palpitations, or a headache. It can in certain instances raise blood pressure and cause irregular heart rhythms and has been linked to some valve abnormalities of the heart, although this is very rare. Other drugs are **Fastin** and **Meridia** and also have similar side effects. There are now new drugs that are being rapidly developed. Many drug companies are eager to exploit the multi-billion dollar market treating obesity. By some estimates, 180 drugs are being tested by more than 70 companies. There are drugs that block hormones produced in the brain. There are other drugs that will block hormones that will regulate appetite in the stomach and intestines. There are still other drugs that regulate hormones that are situated in fatty tissue. Stimulating some of these hormones that are in fat tissue may cause fat to dissolve more rapidly. Other drugs may help people avoid weight gain. The drugs that affect the hormones that are produced in the brain, stomach and intestine all work to decrease appetite and make people eat less. Since there are so many people that are now considered obese in the United States, we should see a rapid increase in the number of drugs coming to market that will help fight obesity. All of these drugs will work by different mechanisms, but mainly by decreasing appetite. Other drugs will help as stated above, by stimulating fat tissue reduction.

A new drug soon to be released is **Acomplia.** This medication has been touted to take weight off and keep it off. It is supposed to work for at least two years. The other diet drugs are only to be taken for a short time period, usually less than six weeks. Acomplia is also effective in lowering cholesterol levels and treating high blood sugar levels. In addition, Acomplia is thought to be effective in helping to stop smoking tobacco. This drug works through a receptor site in the brain that causes cravings. When you take Acomplia, it will block the urges or cravings for food and tobacco. The best thing about Acomplia is that there have been only minimal side effects as compared to the other weight loss pills. We will have to wait and see how this drug works out. It is too early to call it a wonder drug for weight loss.

My ten steps to take to lose weight:

1. Make a **decision**! Take a stand! You need to lose weight and take the right approach. Stay with your decision and realize that it will be a major **commitment**.

2. See your **doctor**. Get a check-up. Have your doctor order some blood work. This should include a lipid profile, TSH, glucose and serum cortisol level. You must be certain that you don't have a thyroid disorder or Cushing's disease - a disorder of the adrenal glands. Also, a complete cardiac work up should be done, if you are about to embark on an exercise program. If you need to, ask about some medication to get you started on your diet program.

3. Avoid foods with **sugar** - don't get that insulin level up. Especially avoid anything with HFCS.

4. Avoid foods with **fats** - this can be stored in the body and is hard to get off. Also, you want to keep those arteries as clean as possible.

5. Keep your **carbohydrate intake** as low as possible. These are hard for the body to metabolize and can be stored as fat. That means stay away from loads of pasta and breads (this is what I was raised on).

6. Keep a log of everything you eat - don't lie to yourself. Do a **calorie count** and find out how much you are really

eating. Avoid the buffet at the local restaurant. Never try to get your money's worth. Don't finish your children's food. When in a restaurant - eat smartly and nothing fried or with butter.

7. **Don't eat at night** - just think of your intestines filled with food. Your body will continue to absorb the food all night long. Go to sleep with an empty stomach - have some fruit or ices before bed.

8. **Do not graze** - you are not a cow, but a beautiful person. Do not eat between meals!! When you are bored or feel unhappy, don't go to the food cabinet and eat chips or other high-calorie, high-fat foods.

9. Start an **exercise** program. This may mean walking or riding a bicycle. You need to do an hour a day of exercise. Get a dog - I walk my dogs three or four times a day. This helps me so much and it is fun. My dogs love it too. I walk them first thing in the morning and then again when I arrive from work and again at night.

Join a gym. Go swimming at the YMCA. Lift weights. Do whatever you enjoy. Try to get as much exercise as possible, even at work. Use the stairs, carry the groceries, park far from your building, whatever you can do to get more exercise and burn calories. Get good walking shoes.

Work out at lunchtime. Eat one half of your lunch before the workout to give you energy. Finish the lunch when you get back and before going back to work.

10. Keep it simple - you don't need special pills or to buy anything from TV or newspaper ads. All you need is common sense and a strong conviction to lose weight. Do not try fad diets or miracle pills. Follow the diets that I have provided and start the exercise programs. Losing weight, dieting, and exercising will be a life-long process. If you can stay with it, there will be many benefits.

5 | ER Training

Experience is a hard teacher, because she gives the test first, the lesson afterwards."
Vernon Sanders Law

There is a marked discrepancy between the quality of medical care that I am delivering today and that during my internship and residency. I did my training in the early 1980s in a hospital in lower Manhattan. Medicine has become so much more sophisticated and of much higher quality, in the last 15 to 20 years.

For instance, a patient named Hector Bambino came in through our Emergency Room. He came in with an upper gastrointestinal bleed. He had been vomiting up "coffee ground" material for the last four to five days. Despite all of his vomiting and inability to eat, he somehow still managed to drink alcohol. Hector was a street person. He lived in the Bowery. Sometimes he slept in a shelter and other times on the street, in a box. When I first saw him, he hadn't bathed in over six months. It was on the last day of my Emergency

Room call rotation and I would be transferring to the Intensive Care Unit the next day. As it turned out, Hector Albino was to follow me through my next rotation. When he came into the Emergency Room he had an intractable upper gastrointestinal bleed. This meant that the bleeding wouldn't stop. A scope was placed down his throat to look at his esophagus, stomach, and the first part of the small intestine. He had what is called esophageal varices. That happens when your liver stops functioning and the blood backs up. It backs up into the lower esophagus where the small blood vessels dilate and sometimes ooze blood. If one actually ruptures, you can exsanguinate, in a short period of time. Once, that happened to another patient of mine. He had esophageal varices and one burst open. A relative found him in his kitchen, on the floor, in a puddle of blood.

The treatment for esophageal varices in 1982, in Manhattan, was ice water saturated with epinephrine. We put a nasogastric tube into the patient (a tube that goes into the nose and is passed down into the stomach), and just pumped in ice water and epinephrine. The theory was that the ice water and epinephrine would make the veins constrict. Hopefully, this would stop the bleeding in the stomach and esophagus. In reality, it would work for maybe five minutes. Here you are with this poor guy vomiting up blood and you are pumping ice water and epinephrine into his stomach, through a tube that is placed in the nose. Not a pleasant thought. Not an attractive sight. Definitely not the place to be, especially if you are the patient or the intern on duty. Every once in a while, the patient would cough up some more blood and that would be soaked with ice water. The blood, instead of being bright red or burgundy, was now diluted to a nice fresh pink. The treatment for esophageal varices, now (in 2004), would be to have a gastroenterologist place a scope down into the deep end of the esophagus and inject something that would sclerose the blood vessels, in the lower esophagus. Sclerotherapy would be performed and that is very effective in stopping the bleeding from esophageal varices. There are newer techniques and medications to deal with this problem, but it still is not that easily treated. Still, even in the present time, esophageal varices can rupture and cause immediate death. However, epinephrine-laden ice water is no longer used. At the present time, it would be considered barbaric.

In any event, Hector Bambino was really a nice guy. We began talking (in between his vomiting up blood that would sometimes come out like a high-pressure hose) and he was funny. He was very accepting of what was happening to him. He was Hispanic and spoke English in a funny way. When he wasn't vomiting up blood in my face, he would crack me up. He would say, "Who gave me that nice bath?" The bath consisted of putting him in the middle of the floor, in a room with a drain in the center. Someone took a hose, someone else squirted some soapy stuff on top of his head and he was hosed down from about 20 feet away. No one could possibly get any closer. After all, he lived on the street and hadn't touched water in over six months.

One time, a homeless person was brought in from the Bowery with a rash on his chest. He came in with a cardiac arrest. It was my job to pump on his chest and do cardiac massage. We were all members of the "code team" and had specific jobs. Mine was performing CPR and pumping on his chest. They probably chose me to do this because I was lifting weights then, and had strong arms. The patient all of a sudden went into cardiac arrest with an arrythmia. I turned around to grab the electric paddles. He needed to be "defibrillated (shocked with the paddles)." I was holding the paddles and about to place them on his chest. When I stared at his chest, the rash had moved to the opposite side of his chest. The rash was migrating. I think I scared the bugs that were causing his rash to the opposite side of his chest. I think I scared them with the electric paddles.

I really tried my hardest not to get infested or infected from any of the patients. However, sometimes I just came home itching. I could not help it. I felt bad for a lot of the patients that came into our ER. They would only show up if they were about to die. It was hard to imagine how people ended up in such a bad situation. This was especially disconcerting as we were so close to Wall Street, the money capitol of the world. Most of the people from the street were really nice. So were the nurses that worked in the ER. It was not infrequent that I saw the nurses slipping the patients some money. They treated the patients with respect and sympathy.

Most of the people that we treated in the ER, at this hospital were indigent. On the other hand, we were the hospital for Wall Street. We would have a homeless guy in one bed and sharing the room would be a Wall Street tycoon. The "money guy" was usually the more pitiful and difficult to take care of. From a Physician's standpoint, I would sometimes rather treat a patient for free, as long as I was treated with respect. It would be so rewarding to help someone that was destitute and in desperate need of medical care. The "money people" (as we called them), created a lot of tension and were always threatening us. It was easy to overpower us then. We realized how little we knew. We were interns and the amount of information that we had to learn was overwhelming. It would take years to become a truly competent Physician. The first days in the ER were very difficult and we really tried hard. We used all of our knowledge and experience to help people. Sometimes, it wasn't enough.

I always tell people to try and avoid teaching hospitals in July. This is when all the interns are fresh out of medical school, and have very little experience. The interns are all starting medical rotations and it is when patients are at their greatest risk. If you get sick in July, try to go to a hospital without interns. *That is unless you don't mind letting the interns learn from your problems.*

Hector Bambino was very fortunate to make it out of the ER. I had poured gallons of ice water mixed with epinephrine into his stomach, via the nasogastric tube. While I was doing this he laughed. He said, "quite a job you have there. Who did you know to get such a great position?" Still, I liked him a lot and it was with a great deal of pride, when I saw him make it out of the ER alive, on his way to the ICU.

6 | Alcoholism and Substance Abuse

*"My grandmother is over 80 and still does not need
glasses. Drinks right out of the bottle."*
Henny Youngman (1906 - 1998)

As I picked up the chart to go into my next examining room, I realized it was someone I knew. It was Sarah, a nurse from the hospital. She was an intensive care unit (ICU) nurse. She had stopped working approximately two or three years ago and became a housewife. She was a very competent ICU nurse, extremely fastidious in her work and replete with experience. If I would go to see a critically ill patient in the intensive care unit, I was always pleased if she was the nurse. She would take good care of my patients. I felt secure when I knew she was the nurse for a patient of mine. We had a good rapport and trusted each other.

As I entered the examining room, I gave her a cursory glance as she was sitting on the exam table. She was in a patient gown. I also noticed that her husband was sitting in the room, in a chair right across from her. She did not look the same as I had remembered her. She appeared more drawn and older than I had remembered, from only two years ago. Her hair was straw-like and her skin was sallow. She had put on a lot more weight, but did not look healthy. It was very apparent that something was wrong. As I walked into the room, she put out her arms and gave me a big hug. It was like she did not want to let go. It was more than a "hello hug" - it was a, I am so relieved to see you and please help me. Her grip was so tight. I said, "What's going on? What brings you in today?" She had never been to see me as a patient before. I was a little uncomfortable at this point and I tried to get everything back to her medical care. Her husband said, "We needed to come to someone that we could trust." I said, "What's up, are you not feeling well?" She replied, "There have been a lot of problems." She was being extremely vague and evasive. So, I turned to her husband and I inquired, "What's the matter?" He replied, "I don't know, I am not sure. I think she is having some type of neurologic problem. She seems to lose her balance real easily and sleeps a lot. She is forgetting things. She used to be extremely competent at taking care of the checkbooks, and now I am finding so much money missing. She does not do the house the way she used to, she has lost interest in a lot of things. My wife never seems to eat. Sarah is extremely forgetful and at times actually goes into rages". He was concerned about her driving. He stated that he was hesitant to leave for work and about leaving her at home all alone. I looked at her and I said, "What do you think is going on?" She responded slowly, "I don't know, I don't know what is happening to me." I asked, "How long has this been going on?" She replied, "at least a couple of years", and her husband interrupted and said that this has been going on for at least five or six years. He added that it has been getting progressively worse, all of the time.

Sarah's husband was a nice guy and seemed genuinely concerned about the health of his wife. He told me that he was an engineering consultant for the government. He had his own firm, and their biggest employer was the U.S. government. He frequently had to go away on business trips. Sarah's husband (I later learned his name is Jason) was almost always at work. He was very driven and his work was the focus of his life. When Jason was not working, he was either golfing or going out to dinner or to other work-related events. Sarah and Jason had two children, both of whom were in the final years of high school. The children were not home much either. They were always studying or in after school games or parties. They were growing up and preparing to go away to college.

I did a cursory exam of Sarah. I looked at her eyes, which appeared to be somewhat more yellow than normal. Her teeth also had a distinct, yellowish, hue. Sarah had developed some pronounced wrinkles in her face, and clearly looked older, than when I had seen her two years ago. Her heart and lungs were clear and her belly appeared to be somewhat protuberant. She looked like she put on some weight, but it was more of what we call central obesity - that is, fat located mainly in the abdomen and not in the arms and legs. Jason stated, "Sometimes her body even gives off a funny odor. Her breath got really bad. All she wants to do is sleep all day. When she awakens from her sleep, she is angry at me. To be honest, you are our last hope. She has refused to go to any other doctors, or to receive any type of medical attention. I do not know what to do with her. You are the first doctor she is seeing in many years." I was surprised at this. I stated to myself, how could someone like Sarah neglect herself her medical care. Obviously she is ill. She must know something is wrong. Jason said," Whenever I suggest we go to a doctor, she just yells and screams at me and I have to leave the house."

At that point, I asked the husband to leave the room to allow me to examine the patient more extensively. Two of the nurses were in the room with me, to assist with the exam. One did an electrocardiogram. The other took vital signs and I asked her to get a blood sugar and urine analysis. I did a thorough exam on her. I noticed that she had a lot of bruising all over her body. I asked her point blank, "Is anybody hitting you or abusing you?" She replied emphatically, "no, nobody is touching me, I seem to be falling and losing my balance a lot." I asked her why does she thinks that is happening, and she replied, "I don't know." She seemed to get mad at me with that answer. I said, "why are you agitated and angry with me and why haven't you received any medical care before today?" This seemed to be a very logical question and she starting getting very angry with me and I backed off. Her breath did clearly smell of acetone, a fruity smell. This occurs when someone goes into acidosis and they give off something called ketones. This means that the body is breaking down certain chemicals, and releasing them through the lungs. Her urine confirmed that she was very acidotic. We then confirmed that she is in fact, in ketoacidosis. I thought she may be a diabetic but her blood sugar was normal. She told me that she did not want any blood work to be done. I again thought this was extremely strange and asked why not. She said simply, "Because I don't!"

I continued my examination of her body, looking at her nails, which appeared to be breaking down. In fact, one of the things I always noted about her was that she always had her nails perfectly manicured. I inquired, "You haven't had a manicure in a while have you?" and she responded, "No, I have been too tired to get out of bed to get it done. I haven't been able to find the time to do things." I asked her to stand, and she was shaky and was not able to stand without assistance. I then decided to go ahead and delve into some further questioning and asked her specifically, are you using any drugs? She replied emphatically, "no I would never do that, I would never use drugs." How is your diet? I asked. She replied, "I don't really feel like eating." I then asked her about alcohol. I asked, "Are you drinking?" "Yes, I am having some wine." she replied. I then asked her exactly how much, and at that point she seemed to let it all out and she began crying. In fact, I could not get her to stop crying. She started to tell me that she drank wine from the moment she woke up until the moment she went to sleep. Her drink of choice was wine. In fact, she only drank Zinfandel, which she got from the local supermarket. She started to tell me how much she would drink. She said that she would go to the supermarket and put the wine in a separate bag. She would sit outside the supermarket and 'down' a whole bottle before she even pulled out of the parking space. When she would get home she would drink another bottle, almost in one gulp. It started out as just a little bit of drinking. She liked the taste and the way it made her feel. She initially started having some wine with dinner or a glass of wine in the afternoon. It just gradually progressed to three to four big bottles of wine everyday. I have to be honest and say that I was flabbergasted at the amount of alcohol that she had been consuming. I was also relieved that this wasn't a case of abuse. I was holding my breath in worry that I would have to call the police and report a domestic violence.

Nobody that I ever knew personally was an alcoholic. I had taken care of street alcoholics, when I was in training in New York City. These were usually street people and I never thought of how they came to be that way. I never thought about street alcoholics or their lives, or their families. Did anyone love them or miss them?

The first alcoholic person I ever took care of was a patient named Hector Bambino. He was a short, funny, Hispanic guy that lived on the streets in the Bowery of New York City. He came into the emergency room one night while I was on call. He had an upper GI bleed and he was literally exsanguinating, from vomiting up blood. In between vomiting his guts up with blood, he asked me for a drink. He laughed all the way to his grave. We were never able to completely stop his bleeding. We tried everything possible, but his bleeding would just recur and start all over again. We pumped his stomach. We would pour ice water and epinephrine through a nasogastric tube into his stomach. This would stop it for a small time and then he would bleed again. We gave him multiple units of transfusions of blood and fresh frozen plasma. Hopefully, this would stop the bleeding. We managed to get him out of the emergency room and to the intensive care unit. The gastroenterologist came in and tried Sclerotherapy. That is a procedure where the doctor would pass a scope into his stomach and try and sclerose his ulcers and esophageal varices. The varices are dilatations of the distal esophagus that would open up and bleed. We would not be able to stop that bleeding. People with advanced liver disease from alcoholism or actually any person with advanced liver disease can develop varices.

I was shocked when I met Hectors sister. She was completely different than her brother. She was pretty, alert, educated and very refined. I expected her also to be a "street person". She was lovely and really cared about her brother. She said the family tried everything and still he would not stop drinking until it eventually killed him. When I signed Hectors death certificate, I was shocked. He was only 35 years old. I thought he was about 60. Why did he drink so much alcohol? I remembered that Hector would only drink wine. He usually had cheap wine that he could get for $1.00 for a huge bottle. Why did he continue to drink, despite the fact that he knew that it was killing him?

There have been several alcoholics that I have taken care of in my medical practice. They all seemed to be such nice people and in fact all of them were very intelligent. They had one serious problem, that is, a disease - they simply could not stop drinking. Why did they continue to do something that they knew was so bad for them? This is what I really wanted to understand.

After further interviews with Sarah and Jason, I learned a lot. When Sarah started to drink, she kept it a secret from everyone. She would drink after her husband left for work and then sleep all day long. When her husband would come home from work, the house was usually perfect and she looked fine. This was all a facade. She tried to keep everything perfect until it was no longer possible. Her personality started to change very gradually. She became less perfect. Sarah would at times become extremely irritable and combative. She would fall asleep during meals and sometimes stay up all night.

Her bills stopped getting paid. She was in charge of paying all the household bills and she stopped doing them. She could not keep track of the invoices and sometimes could not remember where she left her checkbook. She became very deceptive and started having the bills sent to a P. O. Box, so her husband would not realize that they were not being paid. The consequences of her drinking were taking effect. The disease was cunning and baffling, it caused her personality to change. It also made her do things that she would never do, if she were not under the effects of alcohol. She would go to the mall and start to spend money recklessly and excessively. Sometimes, she would come home and not even remember what she had bought. Credit card bills began to pile up. Sarah started a slow decline into her own personal hell. Unfortunately, her whole family and close friends were also drawn into the downward spiral.

She denied drinking and she denied having any problems at all. Basically, she knew that she was powerless over her alcoholism. She would even convince herself that she was not drinking. She had been in constant denial of her alcoholism. Sarah refused to even believe it herself that she was an alcoholic - how could that be? She had everything she could possibly want - why would she give it all away? She made sure that her husband did not see her drink and she managed to keep it a secret from everybody. Many people knew and others looked the other way.

After I had examined Sarah and she admitted her drinking problem, I had a long discussion with both she and her husband. According to Jason, Sarah had always denied being an alcoholic. She had an excuse for all of her problems. If her speech slurred or she fell and hurt herself, she would blame her husband. She said he was too hard on her. One day, she could not get up after falling into a closet at night. Her husband pulled her out of the closet and she fell into the wall. She blamed her husband for hitting her. They both knew it was not true, but she always made him fear he would be culpable for her bruises. Her gait was a staggering and she could not stand up without help. She would scream at her husband and sometimes go into violent rages at him. She told him that if he did not do what she asked him to do, she would call the police and tell them that he was beating her. He was fearful of the situation. He was scared of being arrested and losing his consulting firm. He needed his job and had lots of bills to pay.

Her body was covered with bruises because she kept falling. At times she could not stand without assistance. Everyday, she was drinking more than three bottles of wine and sometimes even exceeded that. She would have at least two bottles before lunchtime. She was severely damaging her liver, and slowing developing cirrhosis. Her platelet count had plummeted to 20,000 (the normal count is about 400,000). When the platelet count is low, bleeding can develop anywhere. You can develop nose bleeding or even just bleeding into the skin with mild trauma. When the number of platelets is down one gets bruises on the skin. Sarah was getting sicker and sicker and she had more and more bruises all over her body. Sometimes, the bruises would appear spontaneously, other times as a result of her falling. She would get severely sick and her brain would not work right. Sarah had delusional thoughts. She felt that everybody was against her and trying to take her away. Her personality changed and she became very paranoid. The worst aspect of her personality changes was that she could not control her rages. The more rages she would have, the further everybody withdrew from her. She would then feel terribly guilty and she would drink even more. This would make her even sicker. She was heading into a downward spiral and would not let anybody help her. This was typical of alcoholism. Also, she brought everybody who loved her down as well.

When there was an interval in her drinking she would become somewhat lucid. At that time she would communicate well with her family and friends. She denied drinking and she denied having any problems at all. She would even convince herself that she was not drinking, a self-delusion common in alcoholics. Her husband, Jason, would suspect that she was secretly drinking at times, however, he did not realize that this was the cause of her problems. He felt that there was something else going on. He would sometimes talk to her and say, "Why are you drinking so much? Why are you doing this? Just stop drinking and everything will be okay." She would reply that she would not drink anymore. Apparently, she believed it. Then, she would actually drink double the amount because of the stress imposed upon her. As soon as her husband would go out of the house, she would start drinking again. She was a "closet drinker". She would drink alone and never in front of other people. Their fighting escalated. He would say, "I don't want you around the children, you are a bad influence, don't drive, don't spend any more money." Apparently, she would go to stores and spend money and not even remember doing it. Her credit card was always out for the taking. Some stores at the mall would call and ask when she would come in again. She would spend huge amounts of money in stores and not even remember buying anything.

She was in "full-blown addiction". Her husband didn't know what to do. He did not understand what was happening to his life. He became angry and resentful. Sarah and Jason would fight. He would say, "Please stop drinking and everything will be okay." Her response would always be, "there is nothing wrong with me, I did not do anything wrong." He would become even angrier. His response was escalating the problem. He should have tried to help her, but he did not understand alcoholism. He did not understand that she had to "hit the bottom", before she could actually get help and get better. He didn't realize that she had a disease and she simply couldn't stop drinking. She couldn't rid herself of the alcoholism in the same way that a person with diabetes could just wish away their disease.

When she came to my office, I realized that she was in alcoholic acidosis. She was physically sick and started to vomit in my office. This is a very severe situation and could actually be fatal. I called an ambulance and sent her to the emergency room. She was admitted to the hospital with acute alcoholism intoxication superimposed on chronic alcoholism and liver disease. I put her in the hospital and gave her intravenous fluids. We would give her vitamins and Librium to prevent her from going into delirium tremens. During the time that she was admitted to the hospital, I spoke to her husband and the patient. We would have long talks. We also invited in a counselor and psychologist, who were both addiction specialists.

There was a lot of blame in the air as to who caused the problem. The fact is that no one caused it; she just had a genetic predisposition to alcoholism. She needed help and unfortunately sometimes you have to get very sick or "hit your bottom" before help will be obtained. She was very lucky that she was able to recover and had no legal problems, at that point. Her children came to visit her and we all spoke at length. They loved their mom and hated to see all the pain that she was going through. They knew their mom was a wonderful person, brilliant, caring, funny and exceptionally smart. They were resentful of her drinking and also didn't understand that this was not a voluntary problem, but was out of her control. They were teenagers and needed their mother to be healthy.

Everybody had always wanted to be around Sarah. The only person in the world that did not see that she was such a wonderful person was, Sarah herself. When she was drinking alcohol, she started to have everything taken away from her. She became sick and started to lose some of her beauty. Her skin yellowed and her hair became straw-like. As she drank more, she became after in her abdomen and she lost muscle tone in her arms and legs. She stopped being funny and was extremely "difficult" to be around. The alcoholism took everything that she adored away from her. She was not able to work or even do housework. She wasted their money and estranged all of her friends and family. She even drove Jason away, the man she loved so much.

She recovered rapidly during this hospitalization. She was then admitted to a treatment plan. She actually went to live in a recovery program. She went into a rehabilitation facility. Unfortunately, she went in and out of this same facility two times. It never seemed to "take". She would say that she was better and wouldn't drink anymore. Jason would believe her and was so happy to bring her home. This was the wrong thing for him to do. He was "enabling" her to continue with her alcoholism.

Sarah reluctantly went into a highly-regarded rehabilitation facility for alcohol and drug addiction for one month of rehabilitation. She did not want to be there. She wanted to be home with her family and she felt that she was creating more of a problem. Sarah was paranoid and felt that she was being abandoned. She was concerned about the cost of the treatment, which was not covered by her insurance. The insurance carrier did not approve this facility as one of their facilities, and thus her husband had to pay it all of out of pocket. That did not concern him, he just wanted her to get well and get her back on her feet. She went into the facility and started receiving rehabilitation treatment. She did not stay the whole four weeks. She only stayed three weeks. She convinced her husband to let her out early. He missed her at home and she seemed to be okay. She said she would not drink anymore and that she was cured. He believed her or at least he wanted to. This facility did not offer the husband any treatment. Jason still had a poor understanding of the nature of alcoholism. A lot of people blamed him for her problem, stating that he wasn't caring enough. He also had been ravaged by her alcoholism. He was in a complete state of depression and did not know what to do. He had to start taking care of things that he was not normally accustomed to. He had to take care of the checkbook, get the family out of debt, take care of laundry, children, schools, as well as get back to work and earn some money. He was in a whirlwind and was becoming depressed himself. When his wife stated that she wanted to come home and everything was okay, he was only too glad to take her out of the rehab facility. The counselors recommended that she stay, however, she did not want to. She said that she had no further desire to drink. She stayed home for one day and then her husband went back to work. Everything seemed to be okay. She said she was just going to stay home and clean and get herself together.

Unfortunately, Sarah's recovery only lasted for a couple of days. She said that she was not going to drink. She had even convinced herself that she was not going to have any more wine. Two days after coming home from the rehab facility, she was shopping at the local supermarket. Sarah decided to just pick up one bottle "just in case". The second she got to the car, she opened the bottle and drank the whole thing down. She was in relapse and her disease was again in full force. In fact, she had only had a "temporary stay" of her addiction and she never really was in full recovery. Sarah only had a temporary relief of her alcoholic intake.

She was now again in full-blown addiction. She did not know what to do and did not understand what was happening to her. When Jason came home, he found some empty bottles and he became irate. He yelled, "what are you doing to our lives, why are you doing this to us? Are you crazy?" Again, he did not have any treatment and did not understand her disease. She was not able to stop drinking as much as a diabetic could willfully stop having a high blood sugar.

Sarah and Jason would fight and argue. He would say, "Please stop drinking and everything would be okay." Her reply would be, "There is nothing wrong with me, I did not do anything wrong." He became very angry. They started to fight and yell again. They started to yell and scream and he decided to go ahead and get a divorce. He could not take it anymore. He didn't know what to do. One night she became very sick and started to vomit uncontrollably. She was dizzy and started to stagger. She again developed alcoholic acidosis and an ambulance had to come and take her to the emergency room. This was about three months after they first came to my office. When she arrived at the emergency room, she again stated that she was an alcoholic, even though she had denied drinking at home. She apparently was self-delusional. She needed more help. She went into the same treatment center, two more times. While she was in the treatment center there was a sense of relief. At least she was being taken care of and was not drinking while in treatment. Jason would be able to get everything organized, talk to the children, get the finances settled, and get the house cleaned and take care of things. Sarah would get treatment and hopefully, this time she would get better.

She would come home and promise that she would not drink anymore and that she was cured. The children were suffering, as they loved their mother very dearly. All of the fighting in the house greatly upset them. Jason finally decided that he needed to get out of the house. However, he was in a dilemma in that he did not want to leave his children alone with Sarah. She was again driving and that also made him very concerned. He was extremely concerned that they would fight and that she would turn violent and that he would be arrested. He was concerned about potential legal problems. He was concerned about the effect that her drinking was having on the children.

Sarah was a beautiful, brilliant, caring and funny person. Everybody had always wanted to be around her. Everyone loved her and admired her. The only person that did not realize that she was such a great person was Sarah, herself. As her disease progressed, she isolated herself even more. She would drink all day and make excuses why she could not go out. When Jason would come home, she would manage to get herself together, shower, do her hair, get the house clean with her housekeeper and everything would seem fine. This would go on for several weeks, until Sarah would become sicker and gradually have to go back into the hospital, because of the alcoholism. One time she developed an ulcer and started vomiting up blood. She was brought to the hospital and required four units of blood transfusion. The gastroenterologist had to go into her stomach and use sclerotherapy on a bleeding stomach ulcer.

Everything was being taken away from Sarah. She became sicker and started to lose her beauty. She lost her sense of humor and certainly her intelligence. Everything around her started to fade as she deteriorated into a dark abyss. She knew what was happening and that the cause was alcoholism. Even though she would deny that alcohol was her problem, deep inside she knew it was. She simply could not stop drinking.

She would wake up in the morning and say "today is the day I am not going touch wine." Then, before 10 o'clock, she had already drunk a whole bottle of wine. Her husband cut up all of her credit cards and took away her car keys. She also was surprised as the checkbooks were taken away from her, and she was given no more money. This made her even more frustrated and wanted to drink even more. The next thing that started to go was her health. She had severe ulcers and recurrent hospitalizations for alcoholic acidosis. She developed severe liver disease. Finally, she became so sick that she had to be hospitalized for an extended period of time.

The situation was deteriorating for Sarah. Jason was at a loss as what he should do. He was becoming depressed and just barely functioning himself. He was lonely and hardly able to work. He tried to take care of his children, but they were always in a bad mood around him and he just left them alone. When Sarah entered the hospital again, for the fifth time, a nurse recommended a new rehab facility. This rehab facility was one that specialized in alcoholics that were professionals. She agreed to go into another rehab center when she got better and was discharged from the hospital. When the time came to go into rehab, she refused. She decided that she wanted to go home and nobody could dissuade her. Of course, she really wanted to go home and drink again. The alcoholic urges were an insurmountable compulsion and obsession. The desire to drink was so forceful that she was willing to give up her beauty, looks, family, children and even her own health in order to drink again. Jason and Sarah continued to argue and the marriage was about to end, if Sarah didn't die first.

Jason could not believe or understand what was happening. He was a prominent consultant, working in his own business. He was making nice money, had a beautiful home, wonderful wife, great kids, and could not understand how this could happen.

Sarah started to drink heavily again. She again waited until she was alone and started to drink bottles of wine, on a daily basis. She was so embarrassed and guilt-ridden. She didn't know why she drank and didn't know how to stop. When she was in rehab, she didn't drink any alcohol. She just bided her time until she was discharged or left early. She knew that she would drink again when she came home. Her alcoholism progressed and it would take so much wine to make her feel good again. Only this time, she became really sick. Her body started to deteriorate and couldn't tolerate all of the alcohol that she was consuming. One day, Jason came home and Sarah was unconscious, lying on the floor. There was a pool of blood around her face. She obviously had vomited blood and then lost consciousness. Jason called 911 and she was brought to the hospital - again. However, this time was different.

In the ER, they told Jason that she was really sick. She was in fulminant liver failure. Her body was in such bad shape that she might die on this hospitalization. She needed a liver transplant if she was to survive. He sat outside the emergency room and just cried and cried. Sarah's liver was in fulminant failure. She was transferred to another hospital where they wanted to do a liver transplant. Her liver was not working at all. Jason was still in a state of shock and disbelief. The children were extremely upset and when they went to visit their mother in the hospital, they could not understand what happened to her. How did things get this bad?

The two children of Sarah and Jason suffered a lot. Their grades were poor and reflected how they felt. They became irate and were unhappy themselves. Their mother loved them, didn't she care about them, didn't she love her children more than wine? These were questions they were asking of their father and he simply did not know the answers. He did not understand the situation himself. Miraculously, Sarah's liver started to work again. She had received intravenous fluids, vitamins and medicine to help stop bleeding, as well as medicine to help ward off delirium tremors (DT's). She did have several episodes where she would become confused and not recognize anybody and hallucinate. This was felt to be from alcohol withdrawal, as well as the liver disease. However, the frequency of the episodes of DT's gradually subsided and she began to regain her health. Her mental status was another question. She appeared very depressed in the hospital. However, no one was sure if this was alcohol withdrawal, alcoholic urges or just being extremely ill.

Her situation gradually improved. She started to slowly regain her health. Her ability to think clearly improved. She became healthier and her color and skin texture started to return to normal. Sarah obtained some texture in her hair and her thoughts became more lucid. Unfortunately, she became sick on several occasions with pancreatitis. This is another problem that you can develop from alcoholism. She developed alcoholic pancreatitis and that sent her back to the intensive care unit on two separate occasions. She became very ill and this was definitely a setback in her medical, as well as her overall healing process. As she began to stabilize medically, she talked to her husband. He stood by her through the whole episode.

Even though Jason felt that he should get out of this situation, he stood by his wife. He considered a divorce so that he could have a normal life. Her alcoholism had been going on for five to six years, by this point. He felt that he should not have to suffer anymore because she decided to drink. Why should he and the children suffer? He felt that she should go live somewhere else, be allowed to drink and eventually die from her medical complications, of the alcoholism. However, he still did love her and wanted his family to be back together, if at all possible. He would do whatever it would require and give her every opportunity available for her recovery. He was truly confused and perplexed as to what to do. There seemed to be no guidance for this situation and he did not know whom to turn to. He was lonely and tired of sleeping alone. He met a counselor in the hospital who advised that he should go to Al-Anon. This is for families of alcoholics. He said, "Why should I have to go to anything, I am not the problem." He did not drink and if she would only stop drinking and return to normal, everything would be okay. He refused to go. He met a counselor in the hospital who told him about another facility for alcoholics.

This facility treated mainly Physicians and nurses. It was a specialty place for drug and alcohol addiction. She highly recommended it. In fact, this counselor (Lori) said that 13 years ago she was addicted to medications and was a patient at this facility. She has been in remission for the 13 years since she was discharged from that institution. She related that this facility does things differently. They do not <u>only</u> treat the patient, but they treat the whole family. She stated that for every alcoholic, there are at least 20 to 30 people that have been affected by the person's addiction. Of course, there are the husband and children, parents, brothers, sisters, neighbors and anybody who came in touch with this person. She stated that things at this time were really raw but Jason should give it a try, at this new facility. He agreed and would do whatever it takes. The counselor made the arrangements and Sarah was transferred to the new rehabilitation program. Jason would give everything he had to get her to stop abusing alcohol. He just wasn't sure what to do. He knew that what had been done before wasn't working.

Sarah was transferred via ambulance to the new alcoholic rehab facility. She did not argue at all. She stated, "I will do whatever it takes to get better." At that time, even though she had been doing better, and her mind was becoming more lucid, she still was under the effects of a physical illness. She had chronic liver disease, chronic alcoholism, brain disease from the alcoholism, as well as lingering effects from pancreatitis and long-term debilitation. Sarah was amenable to anything that would get her healthy. She really did want to stop drinking and return to a normal life, but she simply could not. Upon her arrival in the new facility they took photographs and did some blood testing. They checked her for HIV, which was negative. Her laboratory results were returning to a normal range. She had just spent 4 weeks in the hospital and looked a lot better. However, she still was very ill and suffering the effects of years of alcohol abuse. She was off all medications and eating well.

Upon arrival into the new rehab center, the counselors interviewed Jason. He was required to go through intensive counseling sessions. He said that he really did not need to and he remained angry and feeling frustrated. He was not able to work, his business was failing and his finances were suffering. His relationship with his children and other family members were also strained. He felt that if he could get back to work he would and be okay. He was also concerned about his teenage children as they were starting to "act out" and he was not able to hold everything together at this point. Jason's health started to suffer as well. Even though he worked out regularly, he was not eating properly. He had a loss of appetite and was not sleeping well. He had lost 15 pounds during Sarah's last hospital stay. He missed having an intimate relationship with a woman and was heading into depression himself. He was too strong of a person to admit his own failings and did not want to receive any counseling. Sarah was admitted into the new rehab center and moved into a women's village. They placed her in intensive treatment. The first couple of weeks, she underwent detoxification. Even though she was in the hospital for so long, they felt that she needed to get the remainder of the alcohol out of her system. Since her liver was not working well, the alcohol was cleared very slowly from her body. Sarah was basically getting the alcohol out of her system. She was allowing herself to recover from all of the medical problems that the alcoholism caused. They did give her counseling, good food and put her in with a group of women in similar situations. Jason was not allowed to see her for two weeks. At that time, Jason went home alone, without her. This was actually a relief. He was able to get his home-life managed and speak to his children. The children were actually glad to have the mother out of the hospital, as they did not like visiting her there.

The two-week hiatus from seeing her was clearly a relief for everybody. Sarah threatened to walk out of the rehab facility. It was totally a voluntary stay and they could not force her to remain there. One night they called Jason down to the facility and he talked to her. He said, "If you leave you will die", and that was the truth. If she went out and drank again after having such bad liver disease, pancreatitis, brain disease and kidney shut down - she certainly would die. The potential for bleeding from her stomach ulcers was there and certainly alcohol would exacerbate the ulcers. He convinced her to stay. The counselors at the new facility told Jason that he needed to come to group therapy. That was part of the contract of having her stay in the facility. The family had to get treatment as well. Jason stated that "he did not need any treatment", but he reluctantly went. He didn't want to be near the counselors or any of the other family members of other alcoholics. Just tell his wife to stop drinking and everything will be okay.

One Tuesday night, he showed up to a family meeting. He was surprised that there were about 30 people there. Everybody was sitting in a circle and there were parents, husbands, and wives. Everyone had a severely addicted family member. The facilitator of the group was a psychologist named Cindy. She gave everybody handouts to read. Everybody went around the room and stated their names and how they were feeling that day. Most people said that they were "happy and glad to be there, but were nervous or anxious." When they asked Jason how he felt, he said, "That he was angry, upset and did not need to be in this place." He was openly hostile to the group. The discussion that day was on addiction and how it affects the family. People talked about "tough love" - that is, when the person who is in addiction needs help, the family members shouldn't provide assistance that will enable the patient to continue with their addiction. The alcoholic or addicted client must learn to suffer the consequences of their addiction. Jason wondered how much more could his wife suffer. How much more could his family possibly go through? They were at the end of their rope and needed to get out of this situation. He felt that just divorcing his wife and moving on was the probably the best solution for him and his children. He did not want to go through this recovery process. What did he do to need to be in treatment? He felt that only his wife needed to do that, and he should be left alone and move on with his life.

He spoke to Cindy briefly, and she said, "I am so glad that you have come tonight. We all hoped that you would. You have suffered terribly and we can help you with that. There is no need for you to feel all alone in this." She seemed very sweet and smart, but he really did not want to part of the recovery process. He was very resistant to any type of treatment himself. Cindy understood his anger and his pain, but realized that he would have to come to terms with it himself. He could not be forced into any type of recovery. He departed from the group therapy thinking that this was a complete waste of time. He wanted to go home and get dinner ready, take care of his dogs, take care of his bills, clean the house, and get ready for work for the next day.

The following weekend was for families of the clients and was called "family weekend". Families came from all over the country to visit with the person in the addictions program. This facility was one for Physicians, nurses, and other professionals. In addition, anyone that wanted to be in treatment could come to this facility. People came from all over the country to be admitted to this program. In order to regain your license as a Physician or a nurse, you need to complete several months of the program and be certified that you are free from active addiction and now in recovery. Doctors, nurses, and other professionals came from all over the country to be treated in this program. When Jason came to the meeting, he showed up late. He did not want to be there. He felt that the best treatment for him would be to go for a bike ride or a run, have some good food, go out with friends and enjoy himself. He was very reluctant to be involved in the treatment program. The other center where his wife was treated (5 times) never made him get any treatment. In fact, they never included him in anything.

Jason showed up late and saw that there were over 100 people in the room. There were so many family members there for the family day weekend. There were approximately 30 clients in the program. The rest of the people at the meeting were all family members. People came from all over the country to be with their loved ones who were in the treatment program. They divided all of the people up into three groups, of approximately 35 each. The group of 35 sat in a big circle with the relatives sitting next to the clients. They gave everybody a handout. Both the client and the family had to write down 10 things that you loved about the person and 10 things that you were sorry for. The client would then sit in the center facing one family member and read off 10 things that they were sorry for, followed by the other person doing the same thing. Then they would follow by the 10 things that they loved about that person. The family member would also read off 10 things that they loved about the client. Jason and Sarah listened to the other people. They were the last to sit in the chairs in the center of the group circle. He could not believe what he was hearing out of the other people. People were saying that they were sorry for stealing all their money, getting arrested, ruining their car, not coming to a family member's funeral, stealing children's tuition money to buy drugs, etc. So many people were addicted to so many different drugs - alcohol, heroin, pain pills, ecstasy, methamphetamines, and especially cocaine. People were crying and everything was really "raw". The clients had families that deeply loved them. The things that people loved about each other were their smiles, their kindness, and their ability to be there for them. They loved their relatives and just realized that they had a serious problem - drug and alcohol addiction.

It was Jason and Sarah's turn to sit in the middle of the group. Everybody was looking at them. Sarah was sitting in a chair and facing Jason, with a facilitator standing right over them. Sarah was shaking like a leaf. She was crying and had difficulty getting her words out. She was emotionally distraught. She still looked so ill, from her liver failure and long-term alcoholism. She started to read off her list of things that she was sorry for. She read that she was sorry that he had to go through this. Sarah was sorry for all the suffering that she put Jason and the children through. She was sorry for being an alcoholic. She was sorry for leaving them alone. She was sorry that he had to be alone for all these years. All of her guilt at being an alcoholic came poring out. She left a puddle of tears on the floor. Jason was amazed at how astute Sarah was. He thought she was completely out of touch with reality and was not aware of everything that he and the children had to go through. He really admired her at that point. Sarah was crying uncontrollably at that point and it was difficult for them to go on. Jason read his list to Sarah and hardly remembered what he had written. He remembered saying that he was sorry that he could not heal her. He was sorry that he enabled her to continue drinking without consequence, until she ended up having to try and kill herself. He was sorry that he did not praise her in front of the children. He had been sorry that when things were going bad that he would fight with her instead of just walking out of the house. He was sorry that he allowed her to continue to have credit cards, money and to damage them financially. He did not realize how distraught he was either. He did not realize how low he had sunk in his life. He was also crying and they were both holding each other and had difficulty proceeding.

Next was the "things that I love about you part." They had trouble going on. So much had not been said for so long. They did proceed and she read her list, She loved him for who he was, for his intelligence, good humor, and his kindness. He loved her for being beautiful, funny, and a great person to be around. He loved her for attempting to try and stop drinking and for being in this rehabilitation facility. Jason hardly remembered being in a circle and being around other people. He realized that everybody's eyes were transfixed on them and they had touched a raw nerve in everybody. There was just silence for seconds afterwards until the facilitator came up and said that these people need a lot of prayer. The facilitator (Bobby) was a woman who had been treating people in addiction for many years. She was also a religious person and was an ordained minister. Everybody stopped talking and Bobby asked that everybody start praying at that point. Jason and Sarah were of a different religion, but it did not matter. Everybody was praying to G-d and to a higher power. Everybody was hoping that Jason and Sarah and everybody else in the room would be healed from their addictions, and their families could get back together again.

After that event, Jason started to go to more therapy sessions. He began to accept his own co-dependency and he even started to look forward to going to group therapy. He was able to say all the things that were bottled up inside of him, and this started his healing process. Jason would go to all of the sessions that the facility had available. In fact, this particular center was excellent in that it treated not only the client, but the family of the client as well. Jason urged his teenage children to get counseling and the family went for many counseling sessions together. What Jason started to realize was that the alcoholism was out of Sarah's control. She did not wish to be an alcoholic; she did not even want to drink. Sarah didn't even like alcohol. She just could not stop it. There was a theory that her drinking was of a genetic basis as both her father and mother had some addiction problems.

Jason also realized that he could not help his wife in her alcohol cessation. She had to go through the proper treatment programs and she had to want to stop drinking herself. He realized also that she would not stop drinking until "she hit her bottom". Sarah certainly did hit her bottom; in fact she almost died and lost everything.

Jason enjoyed going to the Tuesday afternoon group sessions, as well as the other sessions. The Tuesday afternoon group sessions were with Cindy, a psychologist, who was an addiction specialist. He learned how to interact with the alcoholic. He learned that he could not help her stop drinking and that he could not stop her from drinking. These were all things that she had to do herself. He learned about his own childhood, his own family and learned a lot about himself. He started thinking about his own behavior and how he interacted with his parents, brothers, children, and wife. He learned what role he played in his own family and why he chose Sarah to be his wife. He thought about his career and activities that he had selected. He had never thought about these things before and going to therapy certainly made him more introspective. Sunday family sessions were with the client and families, whereas the Tuesdays were with the families alone. The interaction between the clients and their families was very interesting. There was a lot of emotion involved and a great deal of love. The parents and other relatives of the clients were always very supportive. They wanted to know what they could do to help. The facilitators always said that what they could basically do is support their addicted relatives and friends and never attempt to make them stop their addictions. That was the job of the client and the addiction center.

Jason became very involved with the facility, and in fact, started to help other people who entered the treatment program. Jason truly believed that the difference between this center and the previous rehabilitation programs were that the family was treated as well. He did not realize how much he was suffering and how much the children needed treatment as well. Without the whole family being treated as a unit, the chances for recovery of the client were minimal. Sarah spent four months in the recovery center and another one year attending there on a regular basis, as an outpatient. At the time of this writing Sarah has approximately two years of recovery. Her liver has completely healed and she has had no further bouts of pancreatitis. Jason and Sarah are living together and their family has healed considerably. They go away on vacations together and everything seems to be quite normal. Sarah still goes for counseling sessions and goes to AA on a daily basis. Jason has stopped going Al-Anon, but goes to regular counseling sessions and is involved with the treatment center. At times, he is still suspicious that his wife will start drinking again, but he realizes he is powerless to prevent her from abusing alcohol. He depends on her treatment to guide them and prays to a higher power that she will never abuse alcohol again. Sarah and Jason have seen many people from the rehab center start using their drugs or alcohol again. They have seen people lose everything including family, jobs and lives. There are many people that went through the recovery treatment and left early or did not stay in touch with the treatment center. Unfortunately, many have died.

There are many ways that you can die from drugs. You can go into organ failure, overdose, or aspirate on your vomit and have respiratory arrest. You could aspirate on your food after falling into a stuporous coma. You could get into a car accident, get arrested by police and lose your life in prison. You can contract a sexually transmitted disease or another disease from using shared needles, such as hepatitis C or HIV. Buying drugs in the street is a very dangerous situation. Alcohol and drugs in our society certainly has reached epidemic proportions. Jason and Sarah and their family have received proper treatment and continue to be in recovery to this day. They are certainly the fortunate ones.

Jason and Sarah are back to their previous lives. They have a wonderful home, children, and are adored by family and friends. Not a day goes by when Jason does not appreciate how far they have come. Sarah and Jason have gone to marital therapy as well as addiction therapy on multiple occasions. They have both expressed what they expect from each other. Jason wants Sarah to continue to get therapy and go to a meeting everyday. He also insisted that she be tested for alcohol at least weekly, for a period of one year. Sarah has consented to that. In exchange, Jason has to keep going to group, as well as family therapy. They continue to go to counseling with a Psychologist, named Ariel. She assists with family members and helps to keep them grounded and to realize what is important in life. Jason still has trouble opening up to Ariel. The psychologist has certainly helped him with his family difficulties and putting his life into perspective. He believes that having his life and family restored is truly a blessing from G-d. However, he still does not like to talk about himself and his ordeal with an addicted wife. Jason is a very private person and would prefer to listen to others than reveal things about him.

As a Physician, I have wondered what my patient that I have treated in the hospital, Hector Bambino would have thought of this type of treatment. I wonder how he would have faired had he been able to get into a rehab center. He was addicted to alcohol. Just like Sarah, he was not able to stop drinking alcohol. My views of him have completely changed since I have seen patients and family go through alcohol addiction and treatment. I think I have learned a lot about alcoholism and drug addiction and that it is necessary for the Physician to intervene right away, in the course of this disease. Hector Bambino might be alive today if we had been able to provide him and his family with a proper treatment center.

This is the 12 steps program to recovery and the basis for the treatment of addiction.

12 Steps To RECOVERY

(Taken from Alcoholics Anonymous, Alcoholics Anonymous World Services, Inc., 1976)

1. We admitted we were powerless over alcohol - which our lives had become unmanageable.

2. Came to believe that a Power greater than ourselves could restore us to sanity.

3. Made a decision to turn our will and our lives over to the care of God as we understood Him.

4. Made a searching and fearless moral inventory of ourselves.

5. Admitted to God, to ourselves, and to another human being the exact nature of our wrongs.

6. Were entirely ready to have God remove all these defects of characters.

7. Humbly asked Him to remove our shortcomings.

8. Made a list of all persons we had harmed, and became willing to make amends to them all.

9. Made direct amends to such people wherever possible, except when to do so would injure them or others.

10. Continued to take personal inventory and when we were wrong promptly admitted it.

11. Sought through prayer and meditation to improve our conscious contact with G-d as we understood Him, praying only for knowledge of His will for us and the power to carry that out.

12. Having had a spiritual awakening as the result of these steps, we tried to carry this message to alcoholics, and to practice these principles in all our affairs.

Truth and Reality

Alcoholism is a disease. An alcoholic cannot wish away the problem in the same way that a person with cancer can wish away that disease. An alcoholic will continue to drink and abuse alcohol, despite all of the serious consequences. An alcoholic will continue to drink even if the family is suffering, and despite all legal, financial, and health problems. Sarah and Jason are Jewish, and I have heard people say, "they didn't know that Jews became alcoholics." Alcohol knows no social or religious boundaries - it is an equal opportunity destroyer of lives and families.

Alcoholism runs in families. There are certain genes that put people at risk for alcoholism. There is also an environmental component to alcoholism. We know that alcoholism is hereditary, but the exact genetics of this disease are not entirely understood. Children of alcoholics need to be watched carefully, for they are at higher risk of developing addictive problems. Again, there are people that have the disease of alcoholism, where nobody in the family has been an alcoholic.

There is no cure for alcoholism. It can only be treated and the treatment is lifelong and should be continuous. I do not believe in alcohol moderation- that is, an alcoholic cannot have a little drink or just a glass of wine with dinner. An alcoholic must not drink anything with alcohol for the remainder of their lives.

Many people can stop drinking with proper treatment. This should be done in a treatment center. While the patient is in withdrawal, medications and special vitamins may need to be administered. This should be done under the care of a Physician experienced in alcohol withdrawal. There is a medication called **ReVia** that is supposed to reduce the craving for alcohol. There is another medicine, **Antabuse** that makes people sick if they drink. I don't feel that either of these medications should be used and they are ineffective in alcohol abuse. Benzodiazepines, especially Librium, is very effective in helping reduce the symptoms and medical problems associated with acute alcohol intake cessation. Benzodiazepines should be used to help with the acute alcohol withdrawal syndrome. An appropriate treatment center will urge the patient to be in treatment for a minimum of three months. This should be in-patient with intensive counseling, individual, as well as group treatment. Some centers will require longer treatment. It may sound like a long time to be in treatment. However, just think of how long the person has been abusing alcohol or drugs. In addition, you must think about the consequences of not stopping. There are several new medications that are available to help prevent a relapse of alcoholism. There is now **Campral**, which is a medication that works in the brain, to suppress the desire to drink alcohol. This drug can be used in patients with liver disease and that is an advantage for alcoholics.

Are certain people and groups more likely to abuse alcohol? Just take a look at any newspaper. How many movie stars and famous people are entering a rehabilitation facility today? These are the lucky ones and the ones that you hear about. Look at how many people you see homeless on the street. Are these bad people - do they want to be that way? In most cases, the street people are simply alcoholics or addicts that didn't have a good backup system. They didn't have funds available for treatment or families that could help them. In many cases, these people had mental illnesses that went untreated as well as other types of drug or substance abuse. I look differently at the homeless now. How did they get there? I find that most alcoholics and substance abusers are very intelligent and decent people. They just have a bad problem that is not consistent with functioning in this society.

What should you do if you have a friend or family member that has drinking problem? If the person that is drinking is unable to abstain from alcohol, they will need help. Hopefully, it will not be the legal system after a DUI. This is usually the case. I have had patients go to jail for many months for a DUI. One patient had severe medical problems and the judge didn't care - he sent the patient to jail for 6 months and the patient became very ill in jail.

Here is what I suggest to do to help alcoholics:

Stop covering up for the person and make no excuses. A person has to hit bottom before they will stop drinking and get help. The family has to stop denying the problem and arrange for an "intervention". If the person doesn't want to stop, there is nothing anyone can do. You just have to take away the car keys and remove yourself financially and legally from the alcoholic.

Be very specific and adamant with your demands - if you want a friend or family member to stop drinking, tell them that they can't be part of your life until they have completed a treatment center's program. In addition, they must go for follow-up care and be tested for at least one year. If they don't listen, remove yourself from their lives. Make certain that your demands are not empty threats - they must be followed through with action.

Get professional help - visit with a counselor at a treatment center and do an " intervention" if possible. If the alcoholic is a family member, you may also wish to consult with an attorney to help with legal advice.

Find strength with numbers of friends - get help from friends and family. Do an "intervention" and get as many of the person's friends and family to assist. Do not try to do it alone - that could backfire. You will also need support for yourself and that brings us to the next suggestion.

Get support and treatment for yourself - you cannot imagine how dealing with an alcoholic has impacted your life and your emotions. After two years of recovery, Jason is still early in his own recovery. He knows that he needs help and will get it when he is ready. Jason, to this day, is extremely grateful that the treatment center where he brought his wife included him in their program. He had a great deal of support from the counselors, as well as the other family members of clients. He tried to go to **Al-Anon** that holds regular meetings for those people in an alcoholic's life. This is crucial, and everybody that has an alcoholic in their lives should go to these meetings. The phone number for the National Drug and Alcohol Treatment Referral Service is 1-800-662-HELP.

Stop drinking yourself - this will help the client go through recovery and make it easier and safer to come home. Remember, when the alcoholic comes home, they will need to change people, places, and things. This means that all of the drinking buddies will have to disappear. No more going to the bar or places where drinking was the main feature. Jason still has a problem going to the supermarket and looking at the Zinfandel, that Sarah used to drink. He has dreams of him walking into the supermarket with a baseball bat and taking it to the shelves of wine.

Summary

The hardest thing about having a spouse or loved-one with alcoholism is knowing what to do. As you can fell from this story, Jason tried everything to get his wife to stop drinking wine. He pleaded, yelled, cajoled, and everything else he knew to get her to abstain from alcohol. It was all to no avail. The truth is that an alcoholic will stop drinking only when the alcoholic wants to stop. Not a second before! If you are a family member of an alcoholic, I would implore you to get professional help as soon as possible. Do not try to intervene yourself. It simply won't work and will only lead to frustration and resentment. Try to protect the children if you can. They will see everything and you should explain that their parent is ill and hopefully, will get better.

If someone you love is having difficulty with alcoholism, call for help. Go to an Al-Anon meeting and speak to people. Go to a rehabilitation center and ask for an "intervention". Have a conference with a counselor and explain the situation. Make certain that the family will get proper counseling. You will need all of the help that you can get. Speak to your doctor and see if they have anything to offer. Meet with your attorney and be certain that all of your financial affairs are in order. Do not allow the alcoholic to drive. Call taxis and if they get behind the wheel, while intoxicated, call the police - you have no option.

Jason wished that he didn't fight with his wife while she was drinking. That was a major error on his part. He didn't know what to do and simply didn't understand the disease and how it affected all of the family members. Somehow, he and his wife made it through this ordeal. He owes so much to the counselors, doctors, and other clients and family members that have helped them. He is so fortunate to have his lovely wife back again. He understands that his wife will always be addicted to alcohol; however, she does not need to be under the effects of alcohol ever again.

7 | Physician Mistakes

"If the facts don't fit the theory, change the facts". Albert Einstein (1879 - 1955)
"Get your facts first, and then you can distort them as much as you please". Mark Twain (1835 - 1910)

Mr. Gary Brandon came to my office for a full evaluation. His Physician had just retired and he decided to come to me. I was very honored that he allowed me to be his Physician, because he was a very prominent man in the town. He was a very religious man and was a minister at one of the largest churches in Central Florida. He was a very lovely man. He had a wonderful disposition, a sunny smile, silvery gray hair, and just an effusive personality. We hit it off immediately. This is surprising considering our different backgrounds.

I came to Central Florida as an internist in 1985. Our backgrounds could not have been more different. I am a Jewish, New Yorker and second generation American. Mr. Brandon's family has been in America probably since the Mayflower landed in Plymouth. He was a deeply religious man with strong moral convictions. He deeply believed in G-d and in helping people. In that, we were similar. He was my introduction to the Christian world of Central Florida. The Christians who reside in Florida are usually very religious. In addition, many of the Christians in Central Florida have a fervid desire to see Israel survive. The local Baptists were some of the strongest Zionists and, in fact, Mr. Brandon had been to Israel seven times. We both agreed that the greatest miracle of our times has been the birth and survival of the State of Israel.

His medical examination was quite easy. He seemed to be in good health. He did not smoke, drink, take drugs, and kept himself trim and fit. He always wore plaid shirts, which were ironed to a crisp and were short sleeved and open to the collar. He wore khakis before they were fashionable. All of his examination was normal, except that there was a little bit of blood in his urine. I told him that I was concerned about this and we should do an evaluation. He told me not to be concerned about it because he was already seeing an urologist, at one of the big clinics in town. He said that he had been completely evaluated and he did not want me pursuing it any further. This happened on several occasions, where he would he would come in to the office; I would do a complete examination, which included a urinalysis. The urine always showed small amounts of blood in the urine (microscopic hematuria).

Gary and I really hit it off. We would talk about many things. I would tell him about my family, how they came to the United States from Russia and from Romania. I told him that my father, served in the United States Army. He had received several medals for distinguished service in the European theater, during World War II. Mr. Brandon was also a World War II veteran and that seemed to make him more affectionate towards me. My father and he had been in battles, in the same theaters of Europe. Mr. Brandon, being a religious man, always seemed to want to talk to me about my Judaism. I told him that I had very strong convictions and that I truly believed in G-d and in the Old Testament. He also was an expert on the Old Testament, and we discussed that. He seemed to remind me of one of the Rabbi's that I had growing up, in that he knew the Bible quite well and would use comparisons of the Old Testament with everyday, contemporary life. I had expressed my feelings regarding the Holocaust to him on numerous occasions. I told him that I was very angry that it happened and that I thought about it frequently. I also expressed that I felt that Jewish people were not appreciated in our society. He agreed with that. He even stated, and it was the first time that I ever heard a Christian person say, that he adored Jews, especially because Jesus was a Jew. I really never tried to talk about religion in my office. Many patients had tried to draw me out and I have always refrained from discussing religion. I always felt that my office should be exclusively medical and one should keep their religious and spiritual feelings to themselves.

I have always felt that being a Physician was truly a religious calling. I love making a good diagnosis, helping people, and providing the most advanced medical care. I certainly was glad to be able to evaluate patients and direct them to the proper medical treatment. This is an honor and it is G-d's work.

It was a blazingly, hot summer day in Florida when I came back from vacation. In mid-July, I took my family on a long needed trip and we drove to South Carolina. We spent a few days in Charleston. We had a lovely time and then came home. I usually dread coming back to my medical practice after vacation, because I never knew what I would find. Sure enough, my premonitions were correct. When I went to the hospital on Monday morning, I heard that for the past week Mr. Brandon had been hospitalized. I called my coverage doctor to find out what was going on and he said "red snappers." Red snappers are a medical term used for tuberculosis bacteria that is found in sputum. It is a laboratory finding, that is, when you do a certain stain called an acid-fast stain and the pathologist or microbiologist sees tuberculous bacillus in the sputum. Mr. Brandon apparently became short of breath while I was away. He went to the Emergency Room. A pulmonologist whom I respect very deeply saw him. He is an excellent lung Physician, and absolutely a gentleman. He is of Latin descent and has the fineness and distinct air about him of someone brought up extremely wealthy. He attended the best schools and universities. He placed Gary Brandon on three different antibiotics for the tuberculosis and placed him in an isolation room, in the hospital.

I went up to see Mr. Brandon on the fifth floor of the hospital and he was in a closed room, not very different from the room where police would interrogate suspects. There was a bed in the room and a large window to look into the hallways and an outside window. He also had a television. Before going into his room, I reviewed the chart. I reviewed all of the Physician's notes, radiologic reports, and there it was staring me in the face, the laboratory report. Sputum microbiology: several acid-fast bacilli seen in the specimen. Well, it certainly wasn't an overwhelming amount of bacilli; it was only a few of them that were seen. It certainly did not say that it was tuberculosis; it was just that there were some bacteria that were acid-fast stained. The chest x-ray was hanging next to the chart. I looked at it, and to my dismay, it was a complete "white out". That means that both lung fields have an infiltrate in all of the lung parenchyma. This means that white blood cells and bacteria have caused a reaction in both lungs and it would be difficult for the patient to breathe. In other words, it looked like pneumonia had invaded both lungs. In addition, Mr. Brandon was walking around with a mask on and no one was allowed to enter the room. I went in anyway. I covered up in a gown, put a mask on, and examined him. He had no fever. He had a little bit of shortness of breath (dyspnea), and a low-grade cough. The cough was non-productive - in other words, a dry cough. He was not terribly ill and had maintained his weight. I had not seen him in a few months, but he certainly did look sicker than he had before. I walked in, "What's going on, my friend?" I asked. "I don't know," he replied. They got me wearing this damn mask and put me on all of these medications." It seemed as if he was questioning the diagnosis, and I didn't blame him. Where would he get tuberculosis from in Central Florida? I did not say anything to him. I kept silent throughout the examination. He had no palpable lymph nodes, no skin lesions, and he just did not appear to have tuberculosis, by my clinical intuition.

I had trained in New York City and have seen droves of patients with tuberculosis. In fact, I have even published an article in the JAMA, Journal for the American Medical Association, about tuberculosis in New York City. I felt that I had a good instinct about this disease, and this case did not "feel like" tuberculosis. What I mean by feel is that you get a certain intuition about patients. I had been practicing medicine since I was a child. I always felt that this was my so-called "calling". I had been volunteering in hospitals since I was a young teenager. I just loved being in the Emergency Room and watching cases come in. I followed doctors around the hospital and especially Emergency Rooms. I had done most of my early training in Maimonides Hospital, in Brooklyn. By the time I was 15-years-old I was going into the Operating Rooms with all of the surgeons. They would let me "retract" in the OR and were always explaining everything to me. My father owned a small diner across the street from the hospital. After I would volunteer at the hospital, sometimes I would go back to my father's store and work the evening shift. One day, I was doing a rotation in Obstetrics and Gynecology at the hospital and had delivered several babies. I came to my father all excited and told him about my day. He still put me to work at the grill. While I was cooking hamburgers on the grill, there was a man sitting at the counter just staring at me. He kept staring and staring and my father said, "Excuse me, sir, why are you looking at my son like that?" The man said, "I could swear that guy cooking the hamburgers just delivered my baby." We all had a good laugh at that one.

Since I had been practicing medicine for so long, I was able to tell who was sick and who was not just by looking at them.

I could see a patient coming into the Emergency Room and tell if he needed attention right away or if his care could be delayed. And that was how I felt about Mr. Brandon. His problem did not seem "infectious" to me. Upon examination, he had no fever, he had no swollen lymph nodes, he did not have an elevated white blood cell count, and his sedimentation rate (a test of inflammation in the body) was not elevated. I spoke to the pulmonologist and told him about my feelings. He said that he was certain that it was tuberculosis, because of the red snappers in the sputum specimen and the x-ray was consistent with tuberculosis. Mr. Brandon had to spend several weeks in the hospital, in an isolation room. He was made ill from many of the antibiotics we gave him. Further, we saw no improvement in his clinical condition or his x-ray. I next saw him in the office, where he was in a much more debilitated state. He was wearing a surgical mask and he said that the pills kept him in a constant state of nausea. He said that he worst thing was that he was not able to see his grandchildren or attend church. I ordered another chest x-ray and it showed a worsening of the "white out". Because of my concern with the diagnosis, I again approached the pulmonologist and encouraged him to do a bronchoscopy.

Mr. Brandon went back into the hospital where a tube was inserted into his lungs and several biopsy specimens were taken. The results of the biopsies revealed no tuberculosis and no granulomas, which is the type of finding you obtain in specimens, in patients who have tuberculosis. In fact, the diagnosis was completely in error. He did have renal cell carcinoma, which is a tumor, which spreads to the lungs from the kidneys. It produces so-called "cannonball metastases". That is large quantities of kidney cancer tissue will actually spread via the blood circulation to the lungs where they become implanted and grow. This can simulate many other pulmonary disorders on an x-ray. Mr. Brandon was informed of the diagnosis. The antibiotics for the tuberculosis were stopped, the mask was removed, and he was sent to an oncologist for further evaluation and treatment. The blood in his urine eventually turned out to be fateful for him. It was a shame that he did not allow me to evaluate it, because I am sure that I would have found out that he had renal cell carcinoma, before it had spread significantly to his lungs.

An urologist previously evaluated Mr. Brandon, and that included an intravenous pyelogram (IVP). That is a test where you receive intravenous dye administered through a vein and then an X-ray shows the kidneys, the ureters, the bladder, and the urethra. He also had a prostate biopsy. This would not have diagnosed renal cell carcinoma, which is a tumor of a kidney (see fig. 7-a). His tumor was sitting outside of an area where it could be seen by an intravenous pyelogram. He would have needed a CAT scan or an abdominal ultrasound to make the diagnosis. Now, whenever I see a patient with microscopic hematuria (blood in the urine), I always order a CAT scan as part of my work-up. At least I have learned something from this case, and I am sure the urologists have as well.

Mr. Brandon succumbed to his illness in a short while. The carcinoma was so advanced that by the time the diagnosis was made, nothing could be done. He did receive a short course of chemotherapy and that was to no avail. Prior to his death, Mr. Brandon thanked me, hugged me, and told me what a great friend and doctor I was. I really appreciated that and that meant a lot to me. Some patients you never forget and he was one that I will always remember.

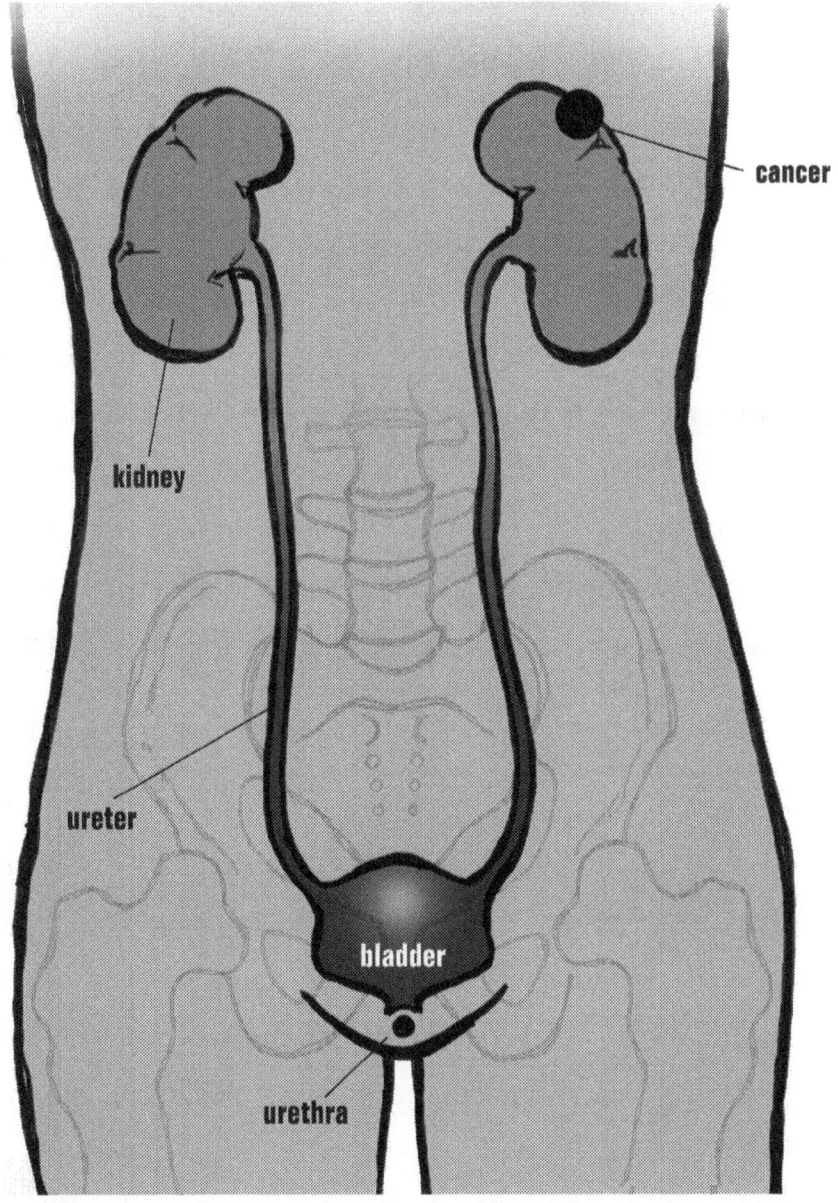

Fig. 7-a. The Urinary system showing cancer of the kidney. Unfortunately, this cancer of the kidney was not seen on the tests that we use to look for this type of tumor. The cancerous growth was on the outside of the kidney and was missed by the radiologic test. It was an unusual place for the tumor to grow.

I did not attend his funeral. I always feel strange doing that as a Physician. People tend to look around and no matter what you did or how you helped someone; they always look at you suspiciously. Sometimes, their death is inevitable and all you can do is palliate their symptoms. Still, family and friends look at you and say, "Is that the doctor who allowed him to die?" They say it like I had a choice in the matter. The only regret I have about Mr. Brandon is that he had to undergo the therapy for the tuberculosis and wear a mask, during the final weeks of his life. If it were known that he had cancer and not tuberculosis, he would have been able to go to church and be with his family. I think that the isolation hurt him more than the disease.

Summary

Mr. Gary Brandon was treated for tuberculosis, when he in fact had cancer of the kidney, which had spread to the lungs. The error in diagnosis was due to obtaining a false lab result. It truly wasn't a Physician error, however, the Physicians were led in the wrong direction because of the laboratory abnormality. Unfortunately, the patient was treated for tuberculosis when in fact he had cancer. He was kept in isolation when he should have been allowed to be with his family. This was not a Physician error, but a false diagnosis. It was not a Physician error in the same sense that removing the wrong leg of a patient or prescribing the wrong medication would be. This was not an adverse health care experience caused by human error, but by the labs, which led the Physicians to believe that the patient had one problem, while he actually had another.

Patients and their families need to be involved in the medical process to avoid errors. If you don't understand your doctor's instructions or explanations, ask your doctor to repeat it in understandable terms. Ask questions until you are sure that you understand everything. The family in this situation could have really questioned the diagnosis of tuberculosis and not accepted it so readily. Of course, the family trusted the Physicians to make the right diagnosis and treat the patient appropriately. However, I do believe it is the family's responsibility to always question Physicians when an unusual diagnosis is made. Communication is the key to providing and receiving good medical care. The communication should be between the family, the patient, and the health care providers. When families take the responsibility for their part in the process, they are more likely to have a positive outcome.

There have been many agencies asking for Physicians to report on a voluntary basis any errors that they encounter. I do not believe that Physicians will voluntarily report errors due to the liability for being considered negligent, and for malpractice claims to occur. However, the incidence of medical errors can be reduced. This can be done by having the family and patient interact with the Physicians and other health care providers. Be certain you understand the prescriptions and how to take them. Ask about the most common side effects of all of your medications and interactions with other meds and foods. Make certain that you tell your doctor about all your other prescriptions, over-the-counter medications, vitamins and herbal or homeopathic products that you are taking. If you are told that you need surgery, be certain to ask your Physician if he has performed that surgery many times before. If you have any concerns about the need for surgery, get a second opinion. Remember, you are the patient and need to be an informed consumer.

8 | Hospital Training

I always knew that I wanted to be a Physician. I knew it from when I was a little child. In fact, I was named after my Uncle Charles, who was a Physician. To be a Doctor was the greatest thing in the world, in my eyes. To help people through science and knowledge was an honor. There was also the high regard that one receives in society. Nothing carried such a mark of distinction in my family or in my community, as being a Doctor. A Physician was a man of high honor, high intelligence, and of course made some money. If you drove a Cadillac, it meant you were a good doctor.

I worked as a delivery boy to an Emergency Room when I was very young. My father owned the restaurant across the street from the hospital. I would frequently bring in food and other items to the hospital. Patients, as well as Physicians and other staff would call into the store and I would bring over the orders. I enjoyed going into the Emergency Room a lot. It seemed so important, so vital, and so full of life. Decisions were monumental and it was where people's lives got saved. I loved the power that the Doctors had and the vital decisions that they made without reservation. They spoke in a language that was their own; their own code. There would always be yelling in the air and doors opening and closing, policeman walking through asking for the Doctor's time. Patients would be lying on stretchers.

One day, I was delivering a meal to the Emergency Room. At this time I was not more than 12 years old. I was walking past a closed curtain. A hand reached out, grabbed me, and pulled me in. It was a Physician, a neurosurgeon. He wanted me to help him. He needed me to hold a retractor. It was an emergency. I looked down at the patient and there was a knife going into his head. The Physician wanted me to help him pull the knife out of the head. That was my first taste of the Emergency Room. There was blood oozing out of the cut from the knife wound. There was a funny and acrid odor in the air. The surgeon placed the retractor into the wound and then placed it into my hand - to hold in place for him. He asked me to tug on it a little bit, so that he could see where the knife was going through the brain. It was my first look inside of a skull and I actually was able to see the brain tissue.

I later started to volunteer at the hospital, even in my teens. I just liked to hang out in the different departments.

Sometimes the surgeons would take me into surgery, for me to retract. I remember my earliest experiences at 14 or 15 years of age, working with a surgeon. He was instructing me about all of the different anatomical features on a particular patient. I was retracting for him on a stool, fully dressed in surgical garb just like the full Physicians. The Surgeons taught me how to suture and I used to help them close the wounds after a surgical procedure. All of this and I was still barely in high school. Remember, things were different then. There were no HIPPA laws, agencies governing Physicians, and most important, there were no malpractice suits or liability for Doctors.

I remember doing a number of procedures, but the one that I found the most difficult at a young age, was to witness a mastectomy. I found that quite difficult and still do not enjoy the thought of that. I think that when I saw a mastectomy it was the only time that I truly looked at the patient's face to see who they were. Other procedures did not bother me at all. I became used to blood and pain and sometimes even death.

I used to do a lot of medical rounds with the Physicians. This was especially during the summer, when I was off from school. I would sometimes work for my Dad and when the store was slow, I would go to the hospital, where everyone knew me, and just hang out with the surgeons and other

Physicians. Sometimes, I did it officially through the Office of Volunteering, but most of the time I just did it on my own. I would sit through decisions made by the surgeons on how to operate and how to treat the patients. Sometimes, I would go down to the Emergency Room and help suture patients and do other types of work around the hospital. I would walk with the internists and other Physicians, while they were on rounds. I would listen to their conversations. Why did this patient develop pneumonia? What was the cause of this patient's heart attack? What are the ten most common causes of splenomegaly? How frequently does Hashimoto's disease occur in teenagers? I listened to them all and then would go read about the different diseases at night.

By the time I was 16-years-old I really knew a lot of medicine. I was probably as competent as some of the Physicians, at that time. When I entered into my internal medicine residency I felt very confident. I felt that I had an excellent clinical sense and a lot of it was just being around patients and Doctors, for a long period of time. A lot of it also had to do with having good common sense, as well. Since I grew up as a street kid in Brooklyn, common sense was required. It was essential for survival.

Later, when I was an intern, I used to moonlight in the Emergency Room at a hospital in downtown Manhattan. I would frequently be the only Physician on-call. I remember one occasion where several people were brought in from a car accident and I had to suture up someone's head, placing 170 sutures in her scalp. This is while administering to many other patients simultaneously.

I remember on one cold wintry evening, I heard over the radio transmitter that there was a gang fight in Chinatown. They were bringing in some young kids who had been shot. The nurses all got ready setting up chest tubes, intravenous lines, and preparing for the incoming wounded. What came next I was totally unprepared for. They happened to bring in 17 young Chinese teenagers. All of them were in varying states of injury. When they brought them into the ER, I was one of the only Physicians there and I knew that the situation was going to be bad. I immediately called for help and the whole surgical team came down. What had happened was that someone went into a Chinese disco and opened fire with a machine gun. I later found out that 17 Chinese teenagers were shot and seven were killed that night. I pronounced six of them dead. Before pronouncing them dead, since they were so young, we tried to do everything that we could. We "cracked their chests", that is, we tried to stimulate their hearts by using direct cardiac massage. We would make a slice through one of the rib spaces with a scalpel. We then put in a rib retractor with a circular handle; it would retract the ribs, exposing the heart and the different organs in the thorax. We would just take our hand and start squeezing the heart in an attempt to get it jump-started. We were unsuccessful in all of the cases. It seemed so unlikely that a young vital teenager would die from just such a small bullet wound. That night I was really heartbroken to see so many young lives snuffed out. You just wanted to pinch them and tell them to get up and get out of there. Others with leg wounds and arm wounds seemed to have made it out alive. That was my first encounter with multiple deaths, at one time. That night has stayed with me for a long time. I guess it is similar to what a young soldier would see in a war zone, where a number of his colleagues would be killed and he would be emotionally traumatized. Maybe that was my initial encounter with so much death. Even though I had seen many patients die in Emergency Rooms before, I had never had so many young and healthy looking teenagers die at one time.

The worst cases to deal with in the Emergency Room were when they brought people in from the Hudson River. Sometimes a fishing boat or a fisherman would find a body in the water. Sometimes they were half devoured by fish. The rule was that they had to be brought in to the Emergency Room to be declared dead. Another funny rule was that we had to get their temperature up to at least 94° F, prior to them being declared dead. That was because someone with hypothermia could be in a state, which would simulate death, but when you normalized the temperature they could be aroused and you could get a heartbeat. It was then our job to try to get these corpses to a higher temperature so that we could finally declare them dead. We would put nasogastric tubes in and sometimes even enemas and pour warm saline into these tubes. We would give them warm IV's if we could ever find a vein to put an intravenous in. It was so obvious that most of these people had been in the water for days, if not weeks.

Sometimes I would put a nasogastric tube in, which is a tube that goes through the nose into the stomach. You would push fluid in and sometimes you would withdraw and out would come different types of fish and artifacts from the water. That water was so polluted that I don't think anyone could have survived five minutes in that water, much less five days. I remember on one occasion where we were doing this and I noticed something on the back of the patient's head. When I looked at it, it revealed that it was a bullet hole. The Hudson River was a great place to dispose of victims of murder. How could someone not think that this was fascinating? I really loved doing that, however no one can understand the smell. There are no words to describe the smell of someone coming in after being dead for several days. You could describe their mottled bluish skin, their fingers were gangrenous, and their noses chewed off by fish, eyes were missing. However, the smell was what always got me. After a while, you do get used to it, but I don't think there is any smell that can compare to the odor of a decomposing body.

There was a lot of crime in the area around the hospital. One day a man was brought in who was found to be having seizures on the sidewalk. They brought him into the hospital when I was on-call one day. In fact, a bunch of passer-bys saw him seizing on the sidewalk and just carried him in, one person holding each limb. They lifted him onto a Gurney. I was the first one into the room. What was strange to me was that he was seizing, biting his tongue, and thrashing all over the table. He was having a generalized seizure. However the strange thing was that he was fully dressed. It was a day of over 100° outside and he was wearing a long coat, hat, and boots. I went to take off his coat so that we could try to get an intravenous into him and give him intravenous (IV) medicine to stop the seizures. When I moved the coat away from his belly, I saw tucked into his belt an Uzi machine gun. That scared me because I was worried that it might go off in the Emergency Room and cause injury to someone. But still, I had to get to the patient and try to get him to stop seizing; otherwise he could die from a cardio respiratory arrest. I took a huge scissors and cut through his sleeve and exposed the patient's arm. I saw multiple tattoos and he was profusely sweating, even on his arm. The hair on his arm was all matted.

A nurse came over to help me and we got an IV in. I gave the patient some intravenous Valium and his seizures stopped. The respiratory therapist came over and put in an oral airway so the patient would stop biting his tongue and he would not swallow his tongue or aspirate and die from suffocation. We got him partially stabilized and we decided to try taking off the rest of his clothes. He was wearing high boots. I reached down and grabbed one boot by its heel and gave a yank. We needed to get him cooled down. As the boot came off, out came the cash. Onto the floor dropped 10s, 20s, 50s, and 100s. They went all over the floor. The same thing happened with the next boot. We all stared and looked at each other.

We were making very little money at that time. My weekly salary was about $300 dollars, before taxes. Figuring that I was working 36-hour shifts, we once figured it out to be about $2 per hour. It was almost slave labor considering how hard we worked and the responsibility that we endured. In any event, the cash looked to be a lot and we were all tempted to grab it all and stick it in our pockets. We knew it was "bad money" though. We knew that if we took it and the money just disappeared, someone would be coming after us. I yelled, "don't touch it", and we simply did not even go near the money. We called in Security and the police came and they counted the money together. What they did with it, I don't know and I really don't care. I just knew that I did not want anything to do with it. I later found out that there was over $50,000 in cash, in the guy's boots. What had happened was that he was dealing drugs on the street and collecting cash. He kept a long coat on to conceal his weapons. He was also sticking the cash into his boots and that insulated him. He got hot, real hot. The more cash he received, the hotter he became. He finally passed out and developed a heat stroke with seizures. It was a scary evening, as I was concerned that one of his friends would come looking for the doctors to try to get the money or the weapons back.

There were a few times that I felt personally threatened by patients. None was more ominous than the "grandpa dump". This usually happened on Friday afternoons. If you were working in the Emergency Room someone would bring their parents or grandparents into the hospital so that they could go away for the weekend. They wanted to discharge their responsibilities to the hospital to baby-sit the elderly relatives. I remember one person who came in with his grandfather. He was a teenager. He had a huge pompadour, tight jeans with very high boots, and a cut-off T-shirt, exposing his large muscles. He was an obvious gang-banger. He brought his grandfather in for me to examine. The elderly man was very pleasant, soft spoken, and gentle. He obviously had no control over this teenager. I asked him what the matter was and he said that he felt fine. I went out to the grandson and asked him why he needed his grandfather to be in the hospital. He told me, "He is sick." I asked what was the matter with him. He told me, "I don't know. You're the doctor, you tell me. He just needs to be here over the weekend." I said, "if there is no problem, I really can't admit him to the hospital without a diagnosis." He came right up to me, about one inch from my nose, and looked me right in the face and said, "are you trying to tell me that you're not going to put my sick grandfather into the hospital?" I looked at the corner of the Emergency Room and I saw about four or five of his friends sitting, waiting for him. They were his gang friends. They did not look like people that you wanted to mess with, especially in view of what I saw a couple of weeks earlier, when so many of the young Chinese teenagers were shot. This was an extremely violent gang and they would not hesitate to use force to get anything they wanted. I said, "no problem. Grandpa actually looks a little ill and he could use an evaluation. We'll get him taken care of for you." Unfortunately, security at the Emergency Room was quite poor then. Anyone could walk in. There were no electronic doors, and the hospital had only one or two security guards for the whole hospital, and they were not manning the Emergency Room. This type of situation, where we had to admit someone to the hospital that wasn't sick, happened occasionally. We used to call them "social admissions." That is, we would admit them either because the patient had no place to go or because our backs were in the corner by the patient's family. I later spoke to the teenager and he told me that he was going to Atlantic City to go gambling and partying with his friends. He couldn't take care of his relative.

We did treat a lot of Chinese patients in the hospital where I trained. The hospital bordered on Chinatown. For the most part, they were extremely nice and respectful. Many times on Sundays, I would get Chinese pastries, which I thought was very nice of them. They would bring me Danish, which I thought was great until I realized that they were made with pork inside and so I did not eat them. The local people used to hate to come to our hospital because we always drew a lot of blood. They would always yell out, "No blood, no blood." That meant don't take our blood. They felt that blood was a sign of their life and wouldn't want any of their blood removed from the body. I could understand this. We certainly did a lot of testing and sometimes did take too much for blood tests. Basically, the Chinese patients came to our hospital when they were ready to die. When the home remedies and local Doctors failed, they would then come to us for medical care. One lady I remember came in with a tumor on her breast that weighed over 50 pounds. How she survived for so long with such impairment, I have no idea. Frequently, they would come in when the situation was too late. The Chinese population believed in a lot of home remedies. When they would get a cough, they would go down to the herbal shop and gets some herbs. Frequently, the herbal- medicine contained contemporary medicine mixed in. For example, when they had a cough a lot of the herbs contained some anti-tuberculosis medications. That is one of the reasons why there was a lot of drug resistance amongst the Chinese population for certain illness, especially tuberculosis. In fact, I had a paper published on this in the JAMA, Journal of American Medical Association, in 1985.

I remember one young Chinese girl who came in very sick. She was so pale and had a fever. We later diagnosed her with aplastic anemia. That is, when the bone marrow has stopped producing any type of cells. No red blood cells, no white blood cells, and no platelets are produced. This poor 14-year-old girl needed to have her blood tested at least once per day to determine if she needed transfusions. She was being treated very aggressively, and at that time we did not have bone marrow transplants available. She always had a crowd of relatives at her bedside. Unfortunately, they were not allowed in the room because her white blood cell count would go down very low, and she needed to be in isolation, to prevent infections. I developed a close relationship with her, as I saw her on medical rounds every day for six months. The poor young thing had spent her whole teenage years in the hospital. When I would walk in, sometimes she would get very scared, because she knew I had to draw blood. She absolutely detested the needles. I tried to be as gentle and compassionate as possible, but I also had a job to do. Sometimes her friends would be in the hallway and I would talk to them. Between themselves they would talk in Chinese and I could not understand one word. And then when they would talk to me you would hear a New York City accent, I found it quite striking the difference between their Chinese accents and their New York Accent. This was similar to my parents speaking in Yiddish and then to have typical Brooklyn accents in English. The Chinese teenagers also assimilated and dressed very American. A lot of the young girls, as well as boys had a lot of tattoos, body piercings, and they would frequently dye their hair. At the time, it was very fashionable to have either blonde hair or pink hair. There were also multiple combinations of the two types of hairstyles. The older generation was always very conservative. They were dressed very simply and always seemed to be suspicious of what we were doing to their relatives. I guess it was similar to my family. The elder members were more like their ancestors, while the children assimilated into the American styles.

Sometimes, even I questioned what we were doing because I was not sure if we were really helping the patients, at all times. Some of our methods and treatments did seem to be a little out-dated, but that was all we knew and we really did our best. The young girl's name with the aplastic anemia was Wang Lee. She was a very pretty and soft-spoken young woman. She had to stay in a room all by herself and she appeared to be getting depressed, as well as I'm sure, felt very ill. I was saddened to learn that she has succumbed to her illness about three weeks after I switched rotations and she was under the care of another resident. In retrospect, she should probably have been in a major teaching hospital, where she could have had a better chance for survival.

There was a lady who was brought in with a bad stroke. She was admitted to my service and she had a dense stroke. That meant that she was not able to express herself. She was not able to talk due to the stroke. We did not know if she was understood us either. She had what was called a "locked-in syndrome". We all believed that she was able to hear us and understand everything, but she simply was unable to move or express herself. This to me was an internal prison and I felt really sorry for her. We tried to give her the best care that we could and I always made sure that she was well provided for. She also had a problem with her temperature regulation. I believe that her stroke affected her hypothalamus, which is the temperature regulation center. Her temperature would go from very low, about 95 to 96° to all the way up to 104 and 105°, in a short period of time. This would alternate several times per day and would change very rapidly. The only way we were able to control her temperature and try to keep it in normal range was by putting her on alternating heating and cooling blankets. That means that when her temperature would go up, the blanket would turn to its cooling effect and cool her down. On the contrary, when her temperature would go down, it would turn on to heating and it would bring her temperature up to a normal range. This seemed to work well for a couple of weeks. Apparently, not only was her hypothalamus temperature regulator broken, but also so was the blanket's. One day, I walked in and the blanket started to heat her when her temperature went up. I took her temperature and it was about 109°. She almost boiled to death. She died the next day from over-heating. Sometimes our equipment would have failures and that could have very serious consequences. I had a bad feeling for that lady when she came into our hospital. Sometimes you know when things just aren't going to go right.

Bill Bradley was one of the best basketball players ever in college. He played for Princeton University. He went on to become a star with the New York Knicks. This was in the 1960s. He was not very fast and he certainly couldn't jump an inch off the ground. But, he was great around the hoop. He would score easily over bigger opponents and always seemed to make an easy basket around the hoop. Someone once asked him how he was able to get around the hoop so well.

He responded, "It is just a sense of knowing where you are." He had that feeling of where the hoop was and where he was in relation to it. I don't know if he had an excellent peripheral vision or he had some other innate talent that many others lacked. That is, what I was talking about is a "sense" of where you are. Some people are just able to see things a lot clearer than others are. Bill Bradley certainly had the sense, and he knew it. It wasn't only around the hoop, though. He later went on to become a Senator from New Jersey and a legitimate contender for the President of the United States. I remember when he was playing the Dallas Mavericks, he was passing by the Alamo and he got so excited. On the team bus, he said to several of the other players, "we're passing by the Alamo" and they hardly looked up. He was jumping up and down that he was seeing a piece of Americana. This is pure American history and he had a great feel and sense for it. His mood was contagious and after he started explaining what was going on, everyone else on the bus got excited. Walt Frazier, a teammate with the Knicks, said, "I wouldn't have even looked up if it hadn't been for Bill Bradley."

Sherlock Holmes was a man of great insight, as well. In his books, he could look at someone for just a few seconds and tell everything about him. He would look at the heel of their shoe and see if it was worn out a certain way. If it was, he knew that the person had been in the military and he could even tell what rank by how much marching they had done. He would look at a button on a shirt and see if it was missing, or if he had a frayed shirt. He would look at creases in the skin to see if they had been in the sun. Stature, posture, dietary status, and in just mere seconds, he could deduce a lot from a person. I had become fascinated by all of the Sherlock Holmes stories and read them continuously through my life. I always believed that I learned a lot about deducing things from people. Subtleties in a person's skin color, texture, and eyes, breathing patterns can all give you clear signs of a person's health. I believe that all Doctors, especially internists, have to have a little bit of Sherlock Holmes in them, to make proper diagnoses. After all, you see so many patients that this happens without thinking about it. I have seen an average of 30 to 40 patients per day for the last 20 years; that is over 100,000 patients, I examined and interviewed. In addition, I have also had to come to diagnoses and make treatment advice. If, after this amount of time, you don't get a feel for what you are doing and a sense of where you are, then you have not learned a lot and didn't hone your instincts. However, I do believe that any Doctor that has been in the business for that long certainly understands what I am talking about and has that skill.

9 | The Big One - HIV

"We do not write because we want to; we write because we have to."
W. Somerset Maugham (1874 - 1965)

>   **O, Lord, what is man that You should care about him,**
>   Mortal man that You should think of him?
>   Man is like a breath:
>   His days are like a passing shadow.

-Psalms 144:3-4

In 1982, I was an intern in a hospital in New York City. I had noticed that several young men were coming in with very unusual infections. One fellow came in with uncontrollable diarrhea. We started him on intravenous fluids and treated him conservatively, until we could get the stool culture back. He was a nice guy and I was not aware that he was gay or homosexual, at that time. We just felt that he had the usual run-of-the-mill gastroenteritis and treated him as such. When the laboratory results came in, it took me completely by surprise. I had expected to see either Salmonella or Shigella bacteria in the stool culture. I was shocked when it came back Isospora and Cryptosporidium in the stool. I had never seen this before, and I asked several of my colleagues, and they never saw it before either. We went back to the medical library and found that these types of parasitic infections usually occur in people who are immunologically suppressed. We went back and examined the patient, and found no evidence of leukemia, diabetes mellitus, or any other type of immunological suppression. An infectious disease specialist came in and treated the patient for these infections. He had no idea why this young man would get this type of diarrhea. Over the next few weeks, I noticed a number of young men coming into the hospital and to the Emergency Room with unusual infections. Most of these young men were coming in with respiratory infections and severe shortness of breath. After cultures were taken from their lungs, we found many of them to have Pneumocystis carinii pneumonia (PCP).

The types of infections that were seen in these young men were all previously unknown and unheard of by my colleagues and I. What was going on here? I sat down in a room and talked with one young man and asked him where he thinks he got this infection. He said he did not know. He told me that he was a homosexual and led a very active gay life in New York City. His name was Peter Vasquez. He was married with two children. He said that in addition to being married with children, he was also an active homosexual. He stated that his wife knew that he was homosexual, but they did not feel that was a problem, as he was not cheating with other women.

Peter was a lovely young guy, very handsome, and personable. He had a good job as a computer programmer. He would sit in the hospital, the oxygen cannula in his nose, receiving Oxygen, and also getting medicine from an IV, located in his arm. He was frequently typing on his laptop computer in his bed. Despite the antibiotics that we were giving him, his situation gradually worsened. His respiratory status deteriorated and I reviewed his chest x-ray. It showed complete "white-out" of both lungs. The infection was expanding rapidly, despite our usual antibiotics. None of us knew how to treat this infection (PCP), as we had never seen it before. Peter was moved into the Intensive Care Unit and was placed on a respirator. He developed respiratory failure. His wife and two young children used to come and visit him every day. They were lovely and did not understand what was going on, and how he could still deteriorate, despite our best treatments. I went to the library and looked up this infection and saw that this also occurred, mainly in people who were severely Immuno-compromised. This means that the patients did not have any defenses against infection. I could not understand why all these healthy young men were coming in to the hospital with Pneumocystis and other unusual infections. Why should their immune systems be impaired?

In the library, the textbooks did not say anything about this. People who would get these types of infections usually had some type of impairment of their normal defense mechanisms. This would occur in people undergoing chemotherapy, where the medicine would destroy their immune systems. Also, people with diabetes mellitus or unusual cancers or on chemotherapy, will get these types of infections. Never before, in all of my training, did I even hear of these illnesses. In one textbook there is a disease called LAV (lymphadenopathy viral syndrome). This occurred mainly in Africa and also in young men. Little did I know that the new name for LAV would later become HIV or AIDS.

As I spoke to Peter more frequently, we became quite friendly. He told me about the sexual culture in the New York City homosexual community. There were a number of bathhouses where young men would go and have sex with multiple partners. Of course, not all homosexual men went to the bathhouses, and not all men that did go, would have sex. However, many did. He told me that, in one year, he had between 500 and 1,000 different partners. I thought, 'oh no, this is going to be bad.' I thought of the potential spread of disease, in this manner.

Peter's condition continued to worsen. We tried to give him several different medications, none of which helped his situation. He was eventually placed on a respirator to help him breathe. He would go in and out of consciousness, and several of his other organ systems started to fail, as well as his lungs. He went into kidney failure and he was started on dialysis. Several of the other interns and residents would come and visit him every day, despite Peter being my patient. I did not understand why they came in so frequently. Several of them would kiss his forehead on the way out. I thought that this was kind of dangerous, knowing the type of infection that he had, and at the very least, that this was unprofessional behavior. We received some special medicine from the Center for DISEASE Control (CDC), for his type of pneumonia. This was a new medicine to treat Pneumocystic carinii pneumonia. This was called Pentamidine. It came via special courier and everybody in the hospital was waiting to see if this medicine would work. Peter received it by injection. We all stood around the bed to see if he would get better almost immediately. Unfortunately, Peter died the next day.

I later left that rotation and went on to do an infectious disease rotation, at New York University. Most of our patients were young men who were losing a great deal of weight, and had all types of unusual infections, ranging from tuberculosis to other types of pneumonia. They had all types of viral illnesses and everybody was rushing around to find out what was going on, and to try different new treatment modalities. Some patients were even coming in with unusual types of malignancies. These were mainly skin malignancies, occurring on the face or legs, and included a large reddish growth, which were quite disfiguring. This is unfortunate because a lot the young men who were coming in with these infections, were extremely handsome and took great pride in their appearances. The type of skin tumors that were growing on these people were later found to be something called Kaposi's sarcoma. I again went and reviewed the literature and found that this occurred mainly in old men. There was no clear reason why young men should get this type of malignancy.

I noticed that a lot of the young men only had their mothers at their bedside. The mothers were usually very aggressive in trying to get their children the best of care. That was very understandable, as their children were so ill. At that time, we started to hear about a disease called AIDS. We later found out that these men coming to the hospital with unusual infections were suffering from human immunodeficiency virus syndrome or HIV. The HIV virus was destroying their immune systems and thus rendering them susceptible to unusual infections. These bacteria and viruses that are usually all around us would not infect people with an intact immune system. On an average night, when I would be on-call during residency, I could admit anywhere from 5 to 10 new patients with AIDS-related infections. This was a terrible tragedy to see men in the prime of their life, usually very intelligent with great futures, to be stricken down with such a horrible disease. I actually became quite alarmed when I thought of how many sexual encounters there were between the young men in New York City. Peter told me that he had sex with over 1,000 different people in one year; just imagine how many people could be infected with this virus. The thought of this was overwhelming and extremely depressing. Not much was known at that time about the transmission of the HIV virus. In fact, when I was studying for my boards I went to a medical lecture given by the Chief of Infectious Disease at New York University. He was the "guru" of infectious disease. He stated dogmatically at that time, that HIV couldn't be transmitted from male to female, but only male-to-male. How wrong he was.

On a subsequent rotation at the hospital, I was in the Emergency Room and one night I admitted Peter's wife. Unfortunately, she came in with HIV infection as well. Subsequently, in later months, both of his children were infected. His little son came in with a particularly disturbing illness. His skin was infected with Staphylococcus and he had something called "scalded skin syndrome". His skin was literally peeling off and was extremely painful. It was impossible to go into his room and look at this young child, in severe distress, and pain. He gradually deteriorated, and both of the children and the wife eventually succumbed to the illness and died. I felt completely traumatized by this whole episode and did not know if I could go on being a Physician. It was only later that I felt some degree of relief, when I found out that there was medicine being developed to treat the underlying AIDS virus. We had been treating only the infections that were due to a patient being infected by the AIDS virus. Now, there are all types of medicine to help treat HIV and it certainly is a much more controllable disease, although a lot still has to be done. Now, there are all different types of protease inhibitors and other antiviral medications, which will be successful in treating the HIV virus, before infections can develop. Our greatest focus in the future will be in the use of real agents as monotherapy either in front-line or induction-maintenance strategies. In other words, there will be medicine that will only be necessary to take one time per day as compared to many of the older medications, which requires a patient to take up to 10 to 20 pills per day. This is great news for HIV patients.

There has been a great awareness amongst sexually active people to prevent the spread of viral and other sexually transmitted diseases.

It certainly was interesting to be on the cusp of a new illness that not only shook America, but the whole world. Unfortunately, so many people died from this illness, including many of the interns that I worked with my first year.

Truth and Reality

There are over 40 million people infected with the AIDS virus worldwide. AIDS diagnoses increased by 2% in the year 2002 as compared with 2001. The most recent increases in HIV infection have been among homosexual men. However, there have also been increases in heterosexual transmission of HIV as well.

There has been a revolution in the treatment of AIDS. The new therapies are extremely effective in combating the progression of the disease. One of the key predictors of treatment success is the stage at diagnosis. At the earliest stages of the disease, there are medicines available to prevent further progression of symptoms. There are an estimated 250,000 people in the U.S. that are HIV-positive, and do not know their status. It is imperative that people get tested early to prevent further transmission of the disease. In addition, it is well documented that early treatment will control a patient's viral load and reduce the symptoms.

Most patients with AIDS are treated by family physicians or internists. This is probably a mistake. Patients who are HIV (+) should be treated by an HIV specialist. The drug regimens are very complicated and are evolving rapidly. An HIV specialist can work in conjunction with an internist, but should be the one determining the best strategy for the patient. The CDC has recently stated that many new groups of patients be tested for HIV. HIV testing should be offered in the following situations:

- Persons that request an HIV test
- Unexplained recurrent infections
- Diagnosis of an opportunistic infection
- Diagnosis of recurrent infections
- Laboratory findings of HIV/AIDS
- All pregnant women
- Signs or symptoms of AIDS (i.e. diarrhea, weight loss, pneumonia)

HIV infection will suppress a person's immune system. This will allow for an infection to occur in the infected person. These infections are called opportunistic infections. Examples of these infections are:

- Pneumocystis carinii pneumonia
- Oral candidiasis (thrush)
- Tuberculosis

- Meningitis

- Toxoplasmosis

- Herpes infections

If you are at risk for an HIV infection, it is very important that you get tested. High risk behavior is having sex with prostitutes, male homosexual intercourse, sharing of needles for drug use, intimate contact with a person that has HIV / AIDS, and receiving multiple blood transfusions. Testing can now be done in the Physicians office. There are also home kits that can be used for testing and can use a small blood sample or even saliva.

If you are (+) for HIV, then further testing will be required. You will need confirmation of the test with an ELISA and Western blot tests. These are more sophisticated lab tests used to confirm the diagnosis. You will need to have a CD4 count and a viral load. This will help the physician to determine the severity and to stage the disease. The CD4 is a measure of your body's white blood cell count. When it is low, you will be at risk for certain infections. Your doctor may need to place you on special antibiotics for prevention of an infection. When the CD4 is below 200/ul, the patient is at very high risk for certain infections. At this CD4 level, the patient should also receive all of the standard immunizations. When the viral load is elevated, you will also be at risk for certain infections and will require more aggressive anti-viral therapy.

The current treatment for HIV infection is very complicated. There are multiple different regimens based on viral load and CD4 counts. The most common medications are protease inhibitors, nucleoside reverse transcriptase inhibitors and non-nucleoside reverse transcriptase inhibitors. These medications should be initiated and followed by an HIV specialist. I will not go into the treatment, at this time, as it is surely to change in the very near future.

The treatment of an HIV-infected patient can be very complicated. The medications all have serious side effects. The physician must know when and how to taper and adjust the medications, for each patient. A patient may also have other illnesses that may impact the effect of the HIV meds. I recently diagnosed HIV in a 75-year-old lady. She has many other illnesses that will affect the treatment of the HIV infection. The other illnesses must be taken into account when she is being treated.

Summary

The AIDS epidemic has had a profound effect on the lives of millions of people around the world. In certain countries in Africa, high percentages of the population are infected with the HIV virus. In the US, there are many that are infected and being treated. In addition, many people are infected and do not know their HIV status. It is so important to be tested so that the spread of this disease can be curtailed, it is also important to know one's HIV status so that treatment can be initiated as soon as possible. There are many new treatments available. An HIV specialist, in conjunction with the patient's family doctor or internist, best administers these. With proper treatment, the HIV-infected patient may be able to live a normal life (think Magic Johnson). It is also so important that we counsel our children on the prevention of HIV infection by avoiding risky activities. I am confident that a vaccine will be developed in the future, to prevent the transmission of HIV.

10 | Afraid of Breast Cancer

" Certain words have always frightened me so much. Cancer, the Holocaust, nuclear attacks - are only words. To overcome your fear of these words, learn as much about these topics as possible. Then they won't be so scary." (Charles Lebowitz, MD - 2005)

Mrs. Athena Hampton came into the office for her regular checkup. Her daughter came with her today and this was somewhat unusual. Athena usually came in alone. She was very private about her medical problems. She always reinforced the need for me to maintain confidentiality regarding her medical problems. So, I felt it was strange that she brought her daughter into the exam room.

Athena was 63 years old and was very healthy. She had slight high blood pressure and was only on a diuretic (water pill). She liked this medicine because she felt that it" helped keep the weight off". Athena was a very pretty woman and was always meticulous in her appearance. She wore the best clothes and was extremely well groomed. Her hair was always perfect and her makeup was done to highlight her fine features. Her husband was a banker and she didn't work. She felt that her job was to take care of him and the family. Now that her children were grown and out of the house, she was active in a lot of charities.

She seemed a little more nervous than usual today. She was chattering and a little too friendly with the staff. She was a very reserved woman, but seemed more effusive today. I had last seen her one-month ago and everything was fine. Her cholesterol was a little high and she wanted to treat it with diet. She was in the office today to have her lipids and blood pressure checked. She did lose a little weight and I thought that was good. She always wanted to be thin, but lately had put on a few pounds. I felt that if she took off a little weight, we could avoid medicine for her high cholesterol.

As I entered the exam room, Athena and her daughter became quiet. Athena was sitting on the exam table. She was in a patient gown that opened to the back. I reviewed the chart as we started some basic talk. She told me that she was feeling well and denied any chest pain, shortness of breath, or any unusual symptoms. I noticed in the chart that her blood pressure was fine and her vital signs were all normal. She had lost 4 pounds from her previous visit, one month ago. The nurse writes on the chart the reason for the visit. Athena said it was personal and she would tell me what was wrong. Her daughter remained in the room and this was the first time that she came in with Athena, for an office visit.

We talked a little bit about her family and how she felt and said that everything was fine. I started to examine her. She became very quiet and placed her hand over the front of the gown. I asked her, "what's going on - there's something wrong, isn't there?" She replied, "I am a little worried. There is a small bump on my right breast." I said, "oh? That is strange. You just had a mammogram six months ago and it was read as normal." I checked the chart just to be certain and the report was there. It was a normal mammogram. I said, "probably nothing to worry about. Let's take a look." I asked if she wanted her daughter to stay in the room during the exam. She said " I would feel more comfortable with my daughter here with me." The nurse also was in the room during the exam. I always feel somewhat uneasy about doing an exam on a female patient with the family watching.

I examined her breasts in fine detail. There was a small, pea-sized nodule in the upper - outer quadrant of the right breast. This is the most common location for a tumor of the breast. I also examined under her arms and around her neck for any other masses. This is to see if there are any enlarged lymph nodes or other signs of spread of a tumor. After the exam, I sat with Athena and her daughter. I told them that I would like to get another mammogram and possibly a biopsy of the small growth. At this point, I had no idea if the lump was serious or not. It could have been a benign growth or something that would be a lot more of a problem. There were no other nodes or lumps. In addition, she just had a negative mammogram and this made me feel that it may have been benign. If it was malignant, then it would be caught very early and this was good. She understood this and seemed relieved to have it out in the open and to get it evaluated.

She went for a mammogram the next day. We had to wait several days for the test results. The mammogram is a special X-ray of the breasts. It requires that two views of each breast be taken. Each view is from a different angle so that the breast can be seen better. Both breasts are looked at for abnormalities. The breasts will be compared with each other. In addition, the previous mammogram that Athena had several months ago will be compared to the new one. The Radiologist will look for changes in the new mammogram from the previous one. There are many things that will be looked for on the mammogram. They will look for calcifications that can sometimes indicate the presence of a cancer. Also, they will look at the area where she feels a lump. This will be checked to see if a density is seen on the mammogram.

Mrs. Athena Hampton called me several times to see if the mammogram was back yet. Unfortunately, it was taking some time to get the results. The waiting was causing her to have a great fear of the diagnosis. The daughter was also calling me several times a day. I reassured them that the second I obtain the results, I would call them. Her fear of having breast cancer was overwhelming. They were starting to panic.

I did receive the results of the mammogram the next morning. It did confirm my strong suspicion that the lump was malignant. I called the radiologist to speak to him personally about the results. He told me that the index of suspicion for a malignancy was very high. The lesion was not there on the previous mammogram. It measured three centimeters, and I said to myself, "it's at least a Stage II breast cancer." However, I also knew that the diagnosis wasn't 100% confirmed.

Mrs. Hampton and her daughter came in the next morning. We sat in my office and talked a little bit. They sat next to each other and seemed to bond with this experience. They were both dressed impeccably and in a similar fashion. Both had button-up shirts with collars. The shirts looked uncomfortable to me, but so do high heels. They had on beautiful skirts and very expensive jewelry. I knew that Athena had her daughter later in life and she doted on her.

I said, "the mammogram looks like it is a mass. We need to do more tests." The daughter replied, "What do you think the lump is?" I told her "I hope it is nothing, but I am concerned. I have arranged for an ultrasound tomorrow morning for further evaluation. This is to see if the mass is solid or just a cyst. We can talk more after that test". I explained that the ultrasound is just sound waves and is done quickly. "We can talk again in 2 days." I felt bad that they had to go for more tests and still not have a confirmed diagnosis. I arranged for the ultrasound. I also explained that if the ultrasound shows the lump to be solid, she would need a biopsy. The daughter asked in a firm but annoyed manner "Why can't we just take out the lump?" I answered," If the lump is solid, then we need to know the tissue type. This is because different cell - types require different treatment."

The next day, the ultrasound confirmed a solid mass and Mrs. Harrison was sent to a surgeon for a biopsy. This was the only way for us to be certain that this was a cancer. The biopsy is done with a needle under local anesthesia. A small amount of tissue from the lump is removed. A Pathologist then looks it at under the microscope. This doctor can discern a lot from the biopsy. The Pathologist can look at the cells and tell what tissue the cancer cells arose from. The cells will also be characterized by how abnormal the cells are (the grade) and whether or not it is invading other tissues. The Pathologist will also test the cancer cells for the presence of certain receptors on the cell surfaces.

Mrs. Hampton had the biopsy and was told that it can take a couple of weeks for the biopsy results to be available. Both Athena and her daughter had a difficult time with waiting for the results. They called me frequently to see if the pathology report had come in. I again informed them that I would call as soon as I had it. They came in to see me for a follow-up. They knew that the report wasn't in yet. They were both extremely distressed about having to wait for the results for so long. Mrs. Hampton's blood pressure was up and she wasn't eating well. I told them that their fears were understandable. She was extremely concerned that she would lose her breast. She felt that this would make her unappealing to her husband. She was more fearful of losing her breast than of actually having a cancer spread throughout her body.

When I was a teenager, I used to deliver food from my father's restaurant to a hospital. When I would go to the operating rooms, the surgeons would invite me in. Sometimes, I was able to even scrub and assist with the surgery. I would usually hold a retractor during an operation. I guess that I was such a familiar face around the hospital, that they allowed me to get involved. They all knew that I wanted to be a Doctor. Nothing really disturbed me in the OR. I was able to see all types of injuries and surgeries. Gunshot wounds, car accidents, blood and gore didn't bother me. The only surgery that I didn't like to watch was a radical mastectomy. The whole breast and part of the chest wall would be excised. The whole chest would be grossly deformed and I thought about the woman waking up to see the results of her procedure.

I told Mrs. Hampton that surgery and treatment for breast cancer has come a long way. There is now breast - sparing surgery that can be performed. Almost all women with breast cancer will have some type of surgical procedure performed. For many women, surgeons can perform a lumpectomy. This means that only the cancer and a little bit of surrounding normal tissue will be removed. Most women now, can have either a lumpectomy or a modified radical mastectomy. Mrs. Hampton seemed to feel better knowing her options and that things may not be as bad as she had imagined. She understood that she may require surgery, however it was the waiting and not knowing that made her anxious. We agreed to wait patiently for the biopsy results. Worrying about what might happen is not of any help and was causing so much unnecessary stress. Most women fear breast cancer. They fear the potential surgery that can lose a part of their body.

It was very important for Athena to look well. She wanted to be attractive in the eyes of others, but especially, her husband.

She was afraid of losing their intimacy and not being pretty to him. She was scared that he would not want to be with her anymore. Athena was essentially petrified that breast cancer surgery would cause her to lose her husband. She was desperate to find out the results and she told me that she was praying all of the time. She was not able to think of anything else, but the results of her biopsy. At least she was being honest at this point, in that she no longer hid her feelings. By expressing her feelings and her greatest fear, Athena was able to cope with the situation. I asked her to come back with her husband, when I have the pathology results and we will all discuss it together. She seemed much more composed and at peace with that decision. She left the office much calmer and walked out with her daughter. It was the first time that I had ever seen Athena in charge and taking control of her destiny. I realized that I didn't know her that well after all.

The Pathology report arrived the next day. It unfortunately confirmed a breast malignancy. The cells taken from the breast biopsy were malignant. She came into the office with her husband and daughter. I informed them of the results and they were all very composed. They had been prepared for this, and took it in stride. Mrs. Hampton asked, "What is the next step?" I told her that she would need to see a specialist - an oncologist. I also wanted her to go to a surgeon. I recommended both an oncologist and a surgeon that were very experienced in the treatment of breast cancer. They left the office and thanked me for my help and I wished them the easiest treatment possible. We scheduled a visit for them to follow up with me in a couple of weeks. Before they left the office, Athena's daughter asked me "how did she get this cancer? How did it happen to her?" I replied, "These are great questions, but first, I don't even know your name. We need to talk some more." She said, "My name is Linda and I am not only concerned about my Mom, but also myself. In addition, I have a little daughter and want to know what our risk of getting breast cancer is." I arranged to discuss these issues with Linda and Athena at a later date. These were critically important issues that needed to be addressed, however the most important thing at this time was to get Athena to a surgeon and have the tumor removed.

Athena went to the surgeon and the oncologist. She was "cleared" for surgery and had it with a few days. All of her blood work and X-rays were normal. I expected her to have an uncomplicated procedure. This was the case, in fact. She underwent the procedure at the regional hospital. They have an excellent facility and do this type of surgery quite frequently. Mrs. Hampton told the surgeon that she wanted to have a breast - conserving surgery. That is, she hoped to have an operation where only the tumor was removed and the remainder of the breast was spared. He told her, " I will do what is possible. However, it depends on what we find when we do the surgery." In other words, if he can remove the entire tumor and there is no invasion into the surrounding breast or into the lymph nodes, then he can do a lumpectomy and spare the rest of the breast tissue. He also told her " we won't let fear have us make the wrong decision. I don't want to do a surgery and then have the tumor recur and have to do more surgery at another time."

I was glad that Athena was now being managed by a surgeon as well as an oncologist, with expertise in breast cancer. This would provide her with the best chance of a complete cure and the possibility of the least invasive surgery. Of course, I knew that her chances for a cure were dependent on the size and spread of the underlying tumor. Athena turned out to be very fortunate. Her tumor was small - 3 cm in its greatest diameter. Of course, this needed to be confirmed by surgery and she would have to have her lymph nodes biopsied to determine if the tumor had spread to them.

Athena underwent the surgical procedure. She was, indeed, very fortunate. The tumor was small and the surgeon removed it easily. The tumor was excised with clear margins. That means that there were no cancer cells in the surrounding tissue. This means that the lumpectomy was the procedure of choice. If the tumor was bigger or more invasive or there was more than one tumor, then she would have had to have a complete mastectomy. Some women actually prefer to have the mastectomy. They are less concerned about the appearance of the breast after surgery. They just want it out and feel that this may give them the best chance for survival and a complete cure. In addition, they can always go for reconstructive surgery at a later date. There is a lot of debate about which is the best procedure - lumpectomy or a mastectomy. The lumpectomy is a much smaller and less invasive surgical procedure and the recovery time is shorter. However, the possibility of a recurrence of the tumor is slightly higher with a lumpectomy than with a mastectomy. For Athena, her breasts were such an important part of her feminine and sexual identity. She felt that her husband might reject her if she did not have her breasts. She was more concerned about what her husband would think than about her chances for survival. However, she was fortunate that she was able to have the lumpectomy and have to deal with the issues of a mastectomy. Athena told me," If the cancer ever comes back - we can always have a complete mastectomy at that time." This made sense for her. I have had other patients feel that they want to have the whole breast removed just to make certain that they have no chance for recurrence. Other patients have had the other breast removed to completely eliminate any possibility of any breast cancer. This is actually happening more frequently in patients that have the genetic risk factors for breast cancer.

Mrs. Hampton was elated that all of the cancer had been surgically removed. She only had a small scar on her breast that was healing nicely. We were still waiting for the whole pathology report to return. This usually takes several weeks. A lot of tests are run on the specimen that was surgically removed. In the interim, we arranged for her to start **radiation therapy**. This process is an effective way to kill any further cancer cells that have been left behind, after the surgery. Usually, only women that have had a lumpectomy require radiation therapy. After a mastectomy, it is not required, except if there is a greater chance of recurrence. For instance, if the section of tumor removed had cancer cells right at the margin of resection.

Radiation therapy is given in a special center, by a radiation oncologist. It is given daily for a few weeks. The reason for radiation therapy is to decrease the possibility of recurrence of the cancer. The benefits are great and there are only minimal side effects. The time to get the radiation therapy is right after the surgery. Mrs. Hampton called me and told me that there was some burning at the site of the radiation. She was also complaining that she felt tired. I told her that these were normal side effects and were only temporary. I called - in some cream to apply to the area of redness on her breast. She completed her course of radiation and was very pleased. Everything was going according to plan. I received her pathology report and asked her to come in and discuss it with me. She came in with her daughter, Linda.

Mrs. Hampton looked well. She was dressed beautifully and her hair and nails were perfect. She got into a patient gown and I examined her. The scar where the lumpectomy was done was barely perceptible. The sutures were on the inside and no suture marks were visible. The breast looked sunburned from the radiation therapy. The cream she placed on the burn helped a lot. I checked her arm for swelling and examined her axilla (medical for armpit) and no masses were palpable. That was all good. She was a little concerned about the final pathology report. She had already received several reports that told her the margins of the tumor were clear of cancer cells. She also knew that the lymph nodes had no evidence of tumor and that was very good. There was no evidence of tumor spread. The only thing left for me to tell her was the results of the special tests. The first test whether there were **estrogen and progesterone receptors** on the cells of the tumor. What this means is if there are specialized sites on the cancer cells for the hormones, estrogen and progesterone. This is very important because it will help us determine if certain medications will work. Many cancers of the breast are dependent on hormones.

Hormones are chemicals that travel through the bloodstream. By blocking the hormones the cells will not be able to grow and may die. Tumors that have both receptors (estrogen and progesterone) have a very good response rate to therapy. In addition, patients with tumors that have both receptors, have less of a chance of recurrence.

Athena's tumor was found to be both estrogen and progesterone receptor positive. Thus, she was started on **Tamoxifen**. This is a receptor- blocker and blocks the effects of estrogen on any tumor cells. Tamoxifen has been shown to prevent breast cancer from recurring or spreading. It blocks cancer cell multiplication. It may also help in preventing any new cancer from developing. Tamoxifen has some other effects - it can help lower cholesterol and strengthen bones. On the downside, it may slightly raise the risk of uterine cancer and blood clots. Recent studies show that **Femara,** (it prevents estrogen from being made in the first place) may eventually replace Tamoxifen. It is now being used after women finish their five-year course of Tamoxifen.

There are other tests in the pathology report that are important for the Physician to look at. However, none of the other tests really influence therapy and are very technical (such as **S-phase analysis and histologic grade** of the tumor).

Mrs. Hampton was really very lucky that she didn't require any chemotherapy. This is reserved for more invasive cancers and those that have spread to other parts of the body (**metastasis**). She was very fortunate that she could get by with a lumpectomy and radiation therapy and subsequent hormonal treatment with Tamoxifen.

I finished my exam with Athena and met with her and Linda. Her husband came by later in the office visit. They were truly grateful for the care and support that my office had provided. Athena told me that her husband had been very close to her and gave her a lot of emotional support during her ordeal. She was scared that he would not want to be with her after she had breast surgery. In fact, as is frequently the case, a husband will become emotionally closer to their wife, during and after treatment for breast cancer.

Athena brought her daughter Linda to the office for a visit, the next week. Linda asked me "how does breast cancer happen?" She also inquired about her risks for getting breast cancer. Both Athena and Linda were scared. They were very concerned that breast cancer might be genetically transmitted. They wanted to do everything to reduce her risk for getting breast cancer. I felt that Linda was scared of this at the times that she came with her mother to my office. She was always challenging me as to why her mother had the breast cancer.

I never did address the risk factors to her previously. I didn't speak to her earlier because she wasn't my patient at that time. The most important issue was to get her mother appropriate treatment as soon as possible.

I told Linda "all women are at risk for breast cancer. If you are very concerned about your risks, there are some things that you can do. If you don't smoke that will help in reducing your risk for all types of cancer. Some studies have suggested that losing weight, exercising, reducing stress levels, and not eating meat, may all reduce your risk for breast cancer." She asked," how does not eating meat lower your risk for breast cancer? I don't see the correlation." She was somewhat hostile and I didn't understand her aggressive behavior to me. I felt that maybe she was scared and transferring some of her fear against me. I attempted to answer her questions to the best of my ability. I told her "sometimes cattle and other animals are fed hormones. When you eat the meat, you may be ingesting some hormones that can increase your risk of breast cancer. I told her there are some things that she can do to reduce her risk for breast cancer. She asked me about the risk of having a mother with breast cancer - "Does that mean I am at higher risk for cancer?" "That was another good question," I told her. I answered, " Recent studies have identified two genes, called **BRCA1** and **BRCA 2.** When mutations occur in these genes, breast cancer may occur". I advised her to get tested for the presence of mutations on these genes. That can be done through a simple blood test. However, I also added " Mutations may occur to these genes at any time and the absence at the time of testing may not mean you have less of a risk. The fact that your mother developed her cancer after the age of 50 means that you may not be at high risk for the disease. The best thing at this time would be to limit alcohol and fat intake, exercise regularly, keep your weight down, and attempt to reduce your stress level as much as possible". I also suggested that she get frequent and an early mammogram. As far as the genetics were concerned, there is still a lot to be learned about the BRCA genes.

If her genetic testing shows that she is at a very high risk for breast cancer, she may wish to start on Tamoxifen. This has been shown to reduce the risk of first time breast cancer. In addition, I have had patients that have had elective mastectomies to prevent the breast cancer. This would require a personal decision. I know of one family where every woman for several generations had breast cancer and the patient took the initiative and had a mastectomy and ovariectomy to reduce the risk of breast and ovarian cancer.

I don't believe that I made Linda feel any better. What she wanted to hear, I was not able to tell her. No one can be free from the risk of cancer and it is something that all of us have to live with. Linda's mother Athena found her own cancer in between her yearly mammograms. She did it with a Breast Self exam (BSE, Figs. 10-a, 10-b). This enabled her to find the lump early and have it removed before it had the chance to spread. This is probably the most important thing that a woman can do to find an early breast cancer.

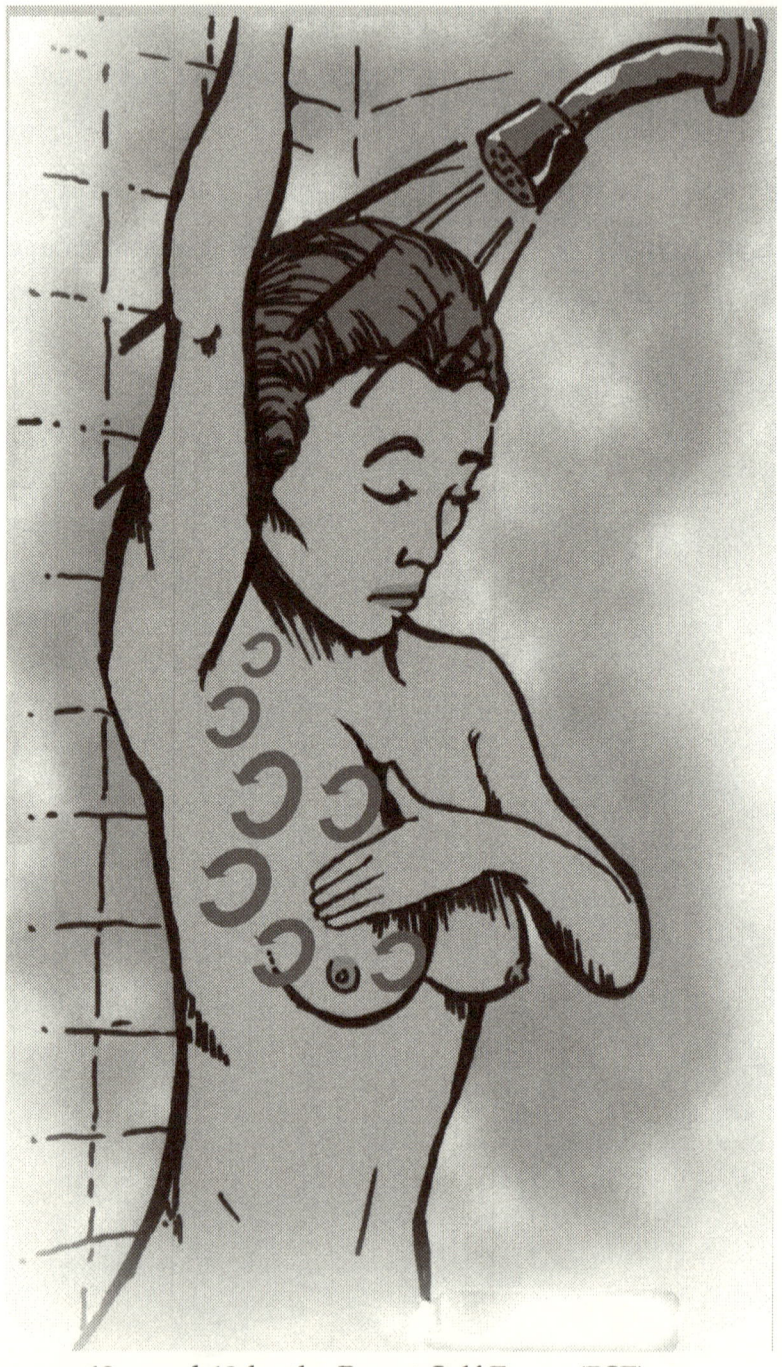

Figures. 10-a and 10-b. the Breast Self Exam (BSE).

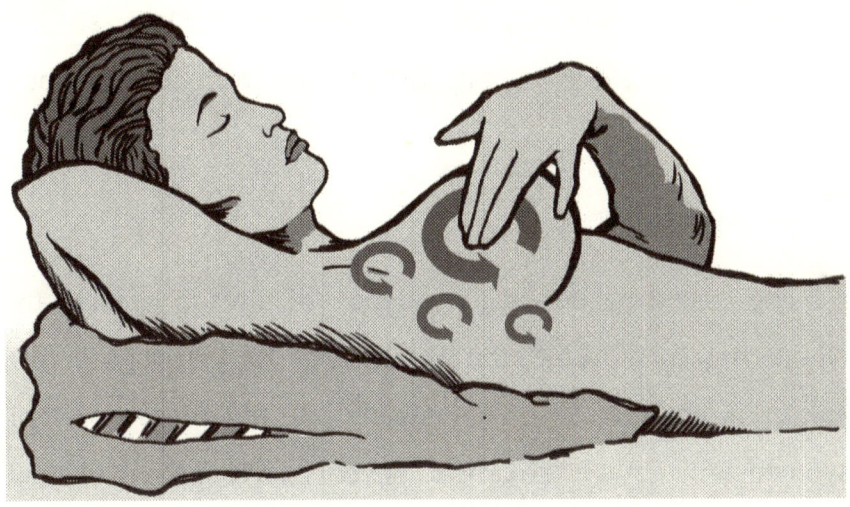

There are many ways to do a Breast Self Exam (BSE). You should do the exam both standing and then again, lying on your back. It is easier to do the exam in the shower, when the breasts are wet. Use circular hand motions over the whole breast. Use you right hand for the left breast and then your left hand for your right breast.

You can also look in the mirror while doing the exam. This is to see if there is any asymmetry between the two breasts. If you notice or feel any new lumps or bulging of the skin, let your doctor know right away. If there is any blood or fluid able to be expressed from the nipples, also let your doctor know. If the nipple has changed or the texture of the skin around the breast has changed, notify your Physician.

You should examine the entire breast on a regular basis. Do the exam softly, but also try to feel deep into the breast tissue. Get used to doing the exam on a regular basis so that you can tell if there are any differences from the previous examination.

Truth and Reality

The statistics on the incidence of breast cancer are staggering. In the USA, the lifetime risk for getting a breast cancer is about 12.5%. That means one out of every eight women will get breast cancer. Seventy five percent of new diagnoses of breast cancer are in women aged 50 and older. The incidence of breast cancer rises with advancing age and is more aggressive in younger women. It is estimated that each year the disease is diagnosed in over one million women and is the cause of death in over 400,000 women. These numbers are truly shocking. It is felt that there is a major environmental component to this disease. Japanese women living in Japan have an incidence 5 times lower than American women. However, Japanese immigrants to the USA, eventually assume the same risk profile as American women.

There are several things that you can do to lower your risk for developing breast cancer. However, you cannot completely eliminate the risk entirely. Probably the most important thing you can do is to do Breast Self Exams. As my patient Athena did, she caught the cancer early. Her treatment was a small surgical procedure followed by several weeks of radiation therapy. She was able to avoid chemotherapy and more aggressive surgery. As for her daughter Linda, she can modify her risk factors, get genetic testing and counseling, and have increased surveillance for breast cancer. As the diagnostic testing gets better, hopefully all breast cancers will be picked up at an earlier stage. This may lead to better and earlier treatment and a better survival rate.

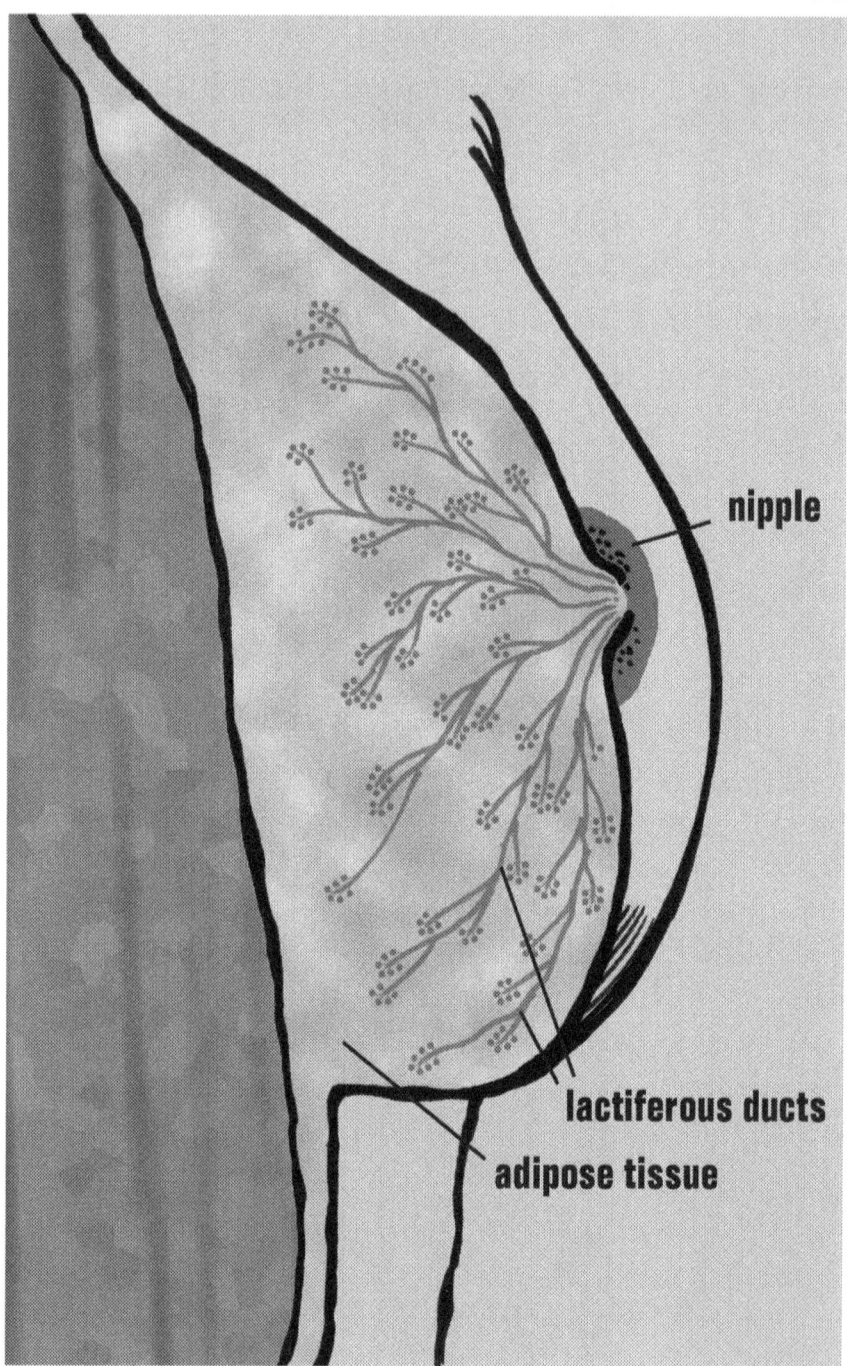

Fig. 10-c. Normal Breast

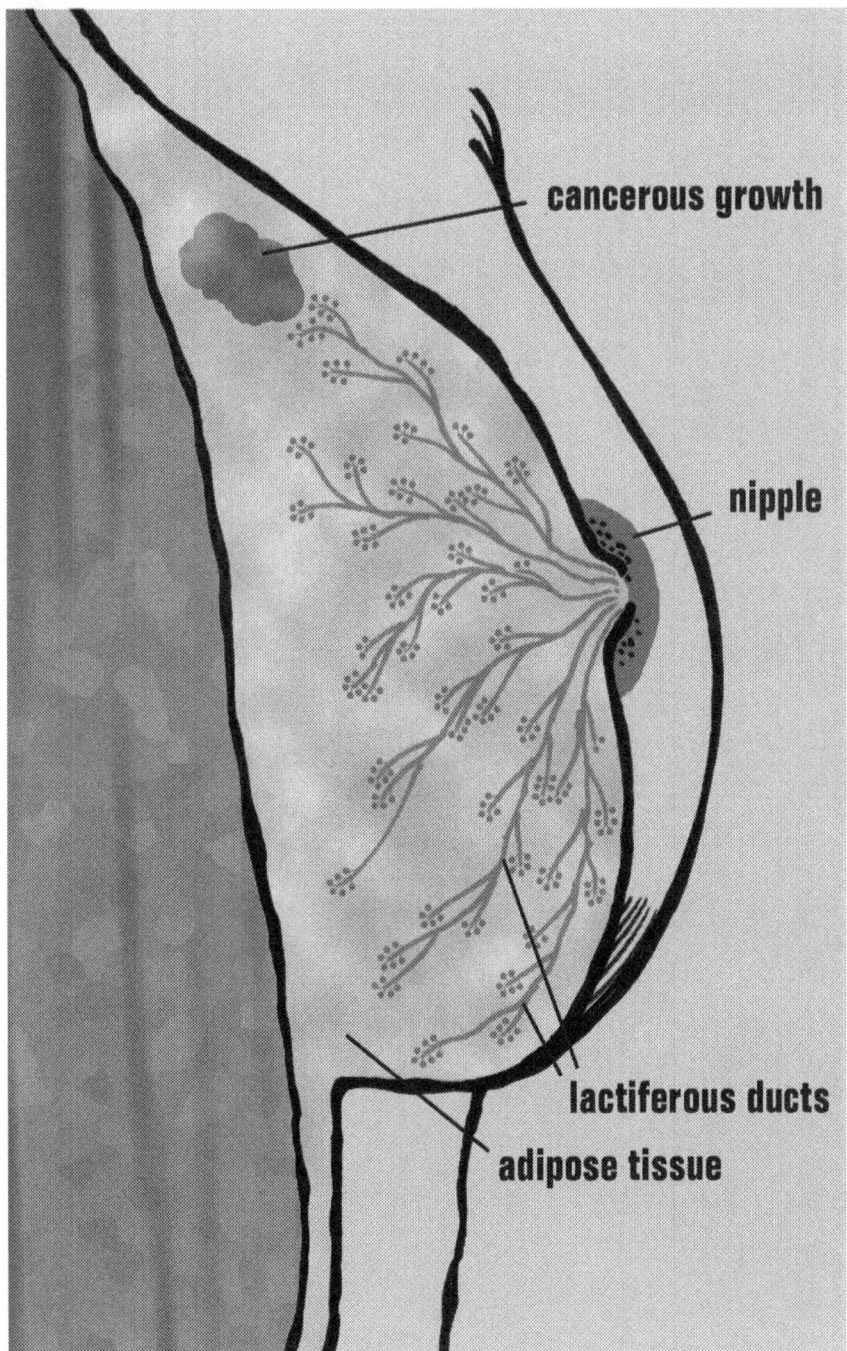

Fig. 10-d. Breast With Cancer

11 | Vitamins and Supplements - Who Needs Them?

"Happiness of a man in this life does not consist in the absence but the mastery of his passions."
Alfred Lord Tennyson (1809 - 1892)

Lillian Hanover walked into the office today. She was usually very cheerful and energetic. She looked different today. Her hair looked grayer and sparser. The skin on her face seemed to have aged very rapidly. I looked in her chart and saw that I had seen her only one month ago. She was complaining at that time that her vision wasn't as good as it had been. I had referred her to an eye doctor to see if she needed glasses. As we age, our vision deteriorates and we need the help of eyeglasses. Lillian didn't like to go to doctors. She believed in home remedies and tried to take vitamins and supplements to avoid medical care. She was a very artistic type of person. She painted and loved music. She never dyed her graying hair and was a free- spirit. She never married and had no family, except for an aging mother that she cared for.

As I entered the exam room, she was already on the exam table. I looked quickly at her file and saw that her vital signs were all normal. It said that she was here because of weakness and fatigue. After some brief chatter, I asked "so, what's going on? How long have you felt ill?" She replied, " I really haven't felt well for a few months. However, in the last month since I saw you, I have become worse." She told me that she was weak and had difficulty getting out of bed in the morning. Her joints were hurting her and she was having headaches. Her hair started to become very coarse and was falling out in places. She noted that her skin was coarser and her lips were cracking and were painful.

I asked her " are you losing weight?" She told me that her weight has stayed about the same." I then interviewed her and examined her over the next hour. There were a million possibilities that could have caused her condition. Everything from a low thyroid disorder to an underlying cancer could cause all of these symptoms. I told her that we need to do some blood tests and further evaluations. As we were talking some more, I saw that her skin was also a little yellow, especially on the palms. I looked at her feet and the soles were also yellow.

I reviewed the chart again and asked her if she ever had her eyes examined and how her vision was. She told me that due to her mother's condition, she had not been able to get to the eye doctor. She said, "Since I wasn't able to get to the eye doctor, I took some mega - vitamins to try and help. I don't think they helped my vision very much." I told her "I think I know what the problem is."

Review the chapter on vitamins and see if you can guess what she did - answer will be at the end of the chapter.

REVIEW of VITAMINS - WHAT THEY ARE USEFUL FOR, WHO SHOULD TAKE THEM AND WHO SHOULD NOT: Vitamins should be a part of staying healthy. Vitamins are special nutrients that your body does not make. You must get it from your food or from supplements.

Everybody needs to have vitamins in their diet. In addition, everybody should be taking vitamin supplements on a daily basis. However, taking too much of a vitamin or consuming too little can both be harmful to one's health. Certain circumstances may require that a person take more of a particular vitamin. Conversely, there are instances in which a person may need to avoid a particular vitamin. The vitamins all have several names, either a letter or their chemical name. Sometimes, they are known by both names. (The following list is taken from the Merck Manual - online edition.)

1. **Vitamin A** - This is also called retinol. There are several types of Vitamin A. The most important type is in the eye's

retina. It is a component of nerve cells that are sensitive to light. It is essential for vision, especially for night vision. Other types of Vitamin A help keep the intestine and lungs healthy and regulate cell growth.

Deficiency: Vitamin A is in all vegetables and meats, eggs and milk. Diseases of the intestine that inhibit the absorption of Vitamin A can cause Vitamin A deficiency. It can also be caused by malnutrition. This occurs in certain areas where diets are deficient in vitamins. The symptoms of Vitamin A deficiency are related to the eyes. One can get night blindness from a deficiency of Vitamin A. The lungs and gastrointestinal tract can be damaged from a lack of Vitamin A and this can lead to major problems - including infections and ultimately death.

Excess: Too much Vitamin A can cause drowsiness and severe headaches and vomiting. If taken over a long period of time, skin disorders will occur and one gets bone and joint pain. The skin will become a yellowish - orange from the excess of Vitamin A (carotene).

Isotretinoin is used to treat acne. This can cause severe birth defects in the fetuses of women that use this during pregnancy. This treatment should be avoided in all potentially pregnant women.

Who Should Take Vitamin A: All people should take the RDA of Vitamin A in a multiple vitamin.

2. **Vitamin B1** - this is also called **Thiamin** - this vitamin is needed for the nerves and heart to work. It is needed to produce energy in cells.

Deficiency: People that go on severe diets may develop B1 deficiency. Also, if you eat only rice, you can get a deficiency of B1. In Asia, the rice is not refined and it keeps the vitamins. Most rice in America is polished and the vitamins are removed. Alcoholics can get a B1 deficiency, if they substitute alcohol for food. Early symptoms of a B1 deficiency are weight loss, abdominal pain, and sleep problems. As the deficiency progresses, beriberi can develop. This is caused by leg pain and nerve problems. It can lead to heart failure and brain problems. The brain disturbances can be very severe and cause memory loss, eye disorders, and eventually death. This is why when we treat people with alcohol abuse or people that have malnutrition; we promptly give them Vitamin B1. If you are dieting intensely, make certain that Vitamin B1 is supplemented.

There are no problems with Thiamine excess. All of the B vitamins as well as Vitamin C are water-soluble. That means that they dissolve in water and any amount not used will be excreted in the urine.

3. **Vitamin B 2** - this is also known as **riboflavin.** This vitamin is essential to produce energy from carbohydrates and amino acids. It also keeps the cells of the lining of the mouth healthy. Sometimes, people with mouth ulcers or irritation are suffering from a riboflavin deficiency.

Deficiency: People that suffer from chronic disorders are susceptible to a riboflavin deficiency. If a person has chronic heart disease, cancer, chronic kidney disease, or diabetes, they are at a risk of a riboflavin deficiency. The symptoms usually start with cracks at the corners of the mouth. The cracks then spread around the nose and mouth. This is called angular stomatitis. The tongue can become purplish and the eyes may be affected. Patients with any type of chronic disease should take supplemental riboflavin.

4. **Vitamin B6** - this is also called **pyridoxine** - This vitamin is very important for the metabolism of fats and proteins. This vitamin is also essential in the production of blood cells.

Deficiency: This can occur in diseases of the intestines, due to malabsorption of the vitamin. Certain drugs will inactivate this vitamin, such as oral contraceptives and some blood pressure medications and INH, a medicine used to treat tuberculosis. Finally, alcoholics are prone to a vitamin B 6 deficiency.

Toxicity: this is possible in the case of an over-ingestion of this vitamin. It can cause neurologic problems and severe dizziness. Thus, it is important to take just the right amount of this vitamin.

5. **Vitamin B12** - this is also called **cobalamin**. This vitamin is necessary for the maturation of red blood cells. It is also needed for nerves to grow and function. This vitamin is normally stored in the liver and would take about 5 years to deplete. Vitamin B12 is absorbed in the small intestine. For this to happen, the vitamin must combine with a protein called intrinsic factor. This is secreted from the stomach. If the stomach is damaged or there is no acidity in the stomach, intrinsic factor can't work. Sometimes, a person can have antibodies against the cells that produce intrinsic factor. This is called pernicious anemia.

Deficiency: This can happen for any reason that the stomach or small intestine is damaged. There can be antibodies against the stomach, lack of acidity, surgery on the stomach. Tapeworms can block the absorption of B12. A strict vegetarian diet can cause a B 12 deficiency, as B12 is only derived from animal products.

The symptoms of a B12 deficiency are first characterized by an anemia. B12 is necessary for the production of mature blood cells. An anemia can cause weakness, fatigue, shortness of breath, dizziness, and the person can be very pale. The next symptoms from a B12 deficiency are related to the neurologic system. Position senses and all feelings of vibration are lost. The person can become confused and eventually a severe dementia can develop. A B12 deficiency can be very harmful to a person.

The only treatment of a B 12 deficiency is Vitamin B12 injections. Oral B12 is of no use if the cause is a disorder of the stomach or intestines, as it will not be absorbed. The shots are usually given monthly for life. Usually the symptoms will resolve with the B12 injections, except if the dementia is severe. That may not get better.

A lot of patients want B 12 shots to " make them stronger and feel better." There is no reason to give these shots, unless the patient has a B 12 deficiency.

6. **Folic Acid** (folate) - This vitamin is necessary for the formation of normal red blood cells as well as other cells.

Deficiency: The most common cause of a folate deficiency is alcoholism. This is because folate is present in fruits and leafy vegetables. Alcoholics are frequently undernourished. In addition, alcohol blocks the absorption and metabolism of folate. There has been an attempt to have folic acid placed in wines and beers. Some companies are adding it to their alcohol - containing beverages.

There are many medicines that block the metabolism of folate and thus are prone to developing a folate deficiency:

Phenytoin (Dilantin)

Sulfasalazine (used to treat ulcerative colitis)

Methotextrate (used for rheumatoid arthritis)

Trimethoprim-Sulfathaxozole (Bactrim - an antibiotic, used to treat urinary tract infections)

There are many other situations that can cause a folate deficiency. Breast-feeding can cause a low folate. Mothers that are breast-feeding or pregnant should be on a vitamin that has additional folate (pre-natal vitamins). People on dialysis need additional folate as well as people that don't eat any fruits or vegetables.

The symptoms of a folic acid deficiency develop an anemia. The first symptom is usually fatigue. They then can become pale, dizzy; develop a personality change, weight loss and shortness of breath. The deficiency can easily be treated with supplemental folate and the anemia should resolve rapidly. Patients with anemia should be tested for a folic acid deficiency, which is usually a simple blood test.

7. **Niacin** (nicotinic **acid**)- this vitamin is essential for the metabolism of many substances in the body. It is needed for the breakdown of fats and carbohydrates.

A deficiency of Niacin is called **pellagra**. This occurs in alcoholics and other malnourished people. It can also happen when there is a disorder of absorption of Niacin in the intestines. Pellagra affects the skin, digestive tract, and brain. The early symptoms of pellagra are weakness, fatigue, abdominal pain, and vomiting. The skin becomes reddened and looks like a sunburn. The rash mainly occurs around the neck, like a necklace. Diarrhea and dementia also occur. In medical school, we learned the 4 D's of pellagra - dermatitis (rash), diarrhea, dementia, and death. This disorder is easily treated with supplemental niacin 200 mg every day.

There is toxicity with Niacin, if one takes too much. This may cause gout, flushing, itching, and liver damage. No treatment is needed, only stop taking the Niacin and the symptoms will resolve. There is no overdose from eating foods with Niacin.

Doctors frequently prescribe Niacin to lower cholesterol and triglycerides. Niacin is very useful in lowering the LDL (bad) cholesterol and raising the HDL (good) cholesterol. Sometimes, the Niacin can cause a flushing of the skin. You can also get skin dryness, diarrhea, and a headache. Taking an aspirin, one half hour before the Niacin tablet, can alleviate these symptoms. Also, the long-acting   (or slow-release) preparations may not cause these problems. Make certain that your doctor checks your liver tests periodically, if you are taking a Niacin supplement.

8. **Vitamin C (ascorbic acid)**- this vitamin is needed for bone formation and helping wounds heal. It also helps the body absorb iron. Vitamin C is also an **antioxidant**. I will talk more about this later. It basically means that it can neutralize substances called free radicals that can be harmful to the body.

A deficiency of Vitamin c is called **scurvy**. Just a few months without Vitamin C and symptoms may develop. Multiple symptoms may occur with a Vitamin C deficiency. These start with weakness and fatigue. Joints and muscles start to hurt and weight loss occurs. The gums become swollen and start bleeding. The teeth may fall out and wounds and infections don't heal. It is estimated that over 2 million sailors died from scurvy in the 1500 - 1800's. The English would take limes on board the ships to eat during long trips at sea. That is why they were called "limeys."

It has been postulated by Linus Pauling, that taking large doses of Vitamin C may prevent the common cold. He also suggested that hyper - doses of Vitamin C might protect the body from other chronic illnesses. Most nutritionists do not believe that large doses of Vitamin C decrease the incidence of the cold or any other illnesses. Vitamin C's cold fighting potential hasn't been documented. Further studies with Vitamin C have not shown this vitamin to be of any benefit in protecting the body from malignant diseases or heart disease or any other chronic diseases. It is of benefit in preventing only the symptoms of a Vitamin C deficiency - scurvy and helps keep the bones, teeth, gums, blood vessels, and other connective tissues healthy. I also like to use 1 gram of Vitamin C daily in patients with chronic urinary tract infections. The Vitamin C is excreted in the urine and makes it difficult for bacteria to grow. This may help in preventing recurrent urinary tract infections. Mega-doses of Vitamin C are not toxic and simply may cause diarrhea and an upset stomach.

9. **Vitamin D** - this vitamin helps the body absorb calcium and phosphorus. These minerals are necessary to build bones. Vitamin D exists in 2 forms. The body makes Vitamin D from sunlight. This vitamin is formed in the skin when the body is exposed to sunlight. It is then absorbed into the bloodstream. Vitamin D is also present in foods such as fish, dairy, and breakfast cereals that have been fortified with Vitamin D. If you don't get outside a lot or live in a rainy area, then you may be deficient in Vitamin D. It will

need to be supplemented in the diet or with a vitamin pill.

Deficiency: with a Vitamin D deficiency, calcium and phosphorus decrease in the blood. The vitamin deficiency may cause **rickets** in children and **osteomalacia** in adults. Both of these disorders are due to a lack of calcium being deposited in the bones. The bones become softer and demineralized. The affected areas of the bones will be painful to touch and fractures may occur.

These disorders are easy to treat with supplemental Vitamin D and calcium.

There are some studies that suggest that low Vitamin D intake is associated with an increased risk of certain cancers. It is thus recommended that everybody take supplemental Vitamin D in a multiple vitamin.

Toxicity: An overdose of Vitamin D can cause an excess of calcium in the blood. This can lead to nervousness, high blood pressure, and vomiting. Eventually, there will be calcium deposits all over the body, especially in the kidneys. Patients may develop kidney stones and kidney failure. The treatment will be to stop the Vitamin D and calcium intake.

10. **Vitamin E** - this is also called **tocopherol**. - This vitamin is called an **antioxidant**. What this means is that this vitamin

protects cells against free radicals. What is a free radical? It's not people against the government. Free radicals are formed from cells that have been attacked and lose their electrons. These electrons attach to other molecules and these attacked molecules lose its electrons. This becomes a free radical and then goes on to attach to other molecules and a chain reaction develops. Excessive damage to cells and tissues may occur if antioxidants are unavailable. Free radical damage increases with age. Vitamins C and E protect the body from the harm of free radicals. They act as scavengers helping to prevent cell and tissue damage by free radicals. Antioxidants neutralize free radicals and prevent them from harming the body.

People with a problem with absorption can develop a Vitamin E deficiency. This is very rare in children and adults. It can occur in newborns. For a long time it was felt that taking large doses of Vitamin E would protect against cardiovascular disease and cancers. The US government did large studies to see if taking these vitamins and other antioxidants would help prevent disease. The studies did not show that taking these vitamins meaningfully decreased the incidence of heart disease or cancer. It is still worthwhile to take these vitamins in a supplement to prevent a deficiency of a vitamin. However, there are **no** recommendations to take supplemental vitamins to prevent or treat heart disease or cancer. Ongoing studies may tell us more about the role of Vitamin E in disease prevention and treatment.

An excess of Vitamin E can be harmful. It can cause diarrhea and weakness and fatigue. At very large doses, it may cause bleeding and other severe problems.

11. **Vitamin K** - this vitamin is needed to make proteins that are necessary to help the **blood clot**. These proteins are essential to control bleeding and thus for the normal clotting of blood. Without Vitamin K, a person can cut himself or herself and the bleeding would not stop.

Deficiency: Disorders of the intestines can prevent the absorption of Vitamin K. Vitamin K deficiency may develop in persons taking certain drugs, including antibiotics and anticonvulsants. We give anticoagulants to people that need to reduce the body's clotting capabilities. **Coumadin** is the main drug that we use to prevent the body from forming clots. This drug acts by inhibiting the action of Vitamin K in the liver. We call this "thinning of the blood", but it really is just preventing clots from forming. People on Coumadin need to be on a special diet and have their blood checked regularly.

The main symptom of a Vitamin K deficiency is **bleeding**. One can get bleeding into the skin, intestines, from ulcers, into the gums, and just about anywhere in the body. A doctor can find a Vitamin K deficiency by measuring a blood test and seeing if the blood clots accurately. The treatment of a Vitamin K deficiency is giving an injection of Vitamin K. Sometimes, if the deficiency is very severe, a blood transfusion of clotting factors may be necessary.

Lately, researchers have found out that Vitamin K is necessary for bone building. If a Vitamin K deficiency occurs, one may get a low bone density and this can lead to osteoporosis. People on Coumadin have to be careful and not take too much Vitamin K. This can affect the ability of the Coumadin to prevent blood clots.

Lillian Hanover wanted to prevent her vision from getting worse. She knew that carotene was important for vision. Lillian took excessive doses of carotene, which is converted to Vitamin A. Excessive doses of carotene causes the skin to become yellow, especially on the palms and soles. It also causes the hair to become sparse (alopecia) and coarse. The skin will become dry and rough and one gets cracking around the lips and face. Headaches develop and people become very weak and fatigued. After we figured out what was going on, Lillian stopped all of her vitamins for a while. Her symptoms resolved, the headaches went away and the skin became normal. This shows the importance of taking the right amount of vitamins and how harmful an excessive dose can be. Oh - she did go to the eye doctor, and looks great in her new glasses.

12 | Syndrome X - What Is This and Why Should We Be Concerned?

"If everything seems to be going so well, then we must have overlooked something."
Stephen Wright, Comedian - 2005

Mr. Thomas Wilkens came to me for an initial office visit. It was winter up north and the snowbirds were coming to Florida. They were also bringing their medical problems with them. Mr. Wilkens is an artist. Apparently, he is a famous artist in the wildlife art world. He does sculptures and paintings of wildlife - ducks, deer, bears, fish, and other outdoor scenes. His work probably adorns the offices of workers who really wish they were outside. I know very little about art. However, I actually had some of his paintings in my home. His work can actually make you feel as if you are in the snow, following a deer. It makes you forget that you are doing paperwork in an office. For some reason, his fish and duck paintings find their way into lawyers' offices.

Since I had never seen him, I was surprised by his appearance. I expected a Grizzly Adams or the rugged, naturalist type. In my mind, he was an athletic outdoorsman who would wrestle with bears and lions. Instead, he was about 5′6″ and weighed over 300 pounds. He had a bagful of medications. He emptied the bag on a table in the exam room for me to see them. We locked eyes and he was ready to give me some grief. " Take these pills and tell me what I need and don't need. I am sick of taking all of the medications. They are making me sick." I replied and stuck out my hand - " Hi, my name is Dr. Lebowitz and I am pleased to meet you. Let's start at the beginning and go through the meds and see what's up. Is that okay?" He replied, " fair enough".

He attempted to take control of the encounter, but I had to put up my boundary. I was the Physician and it was my advice and knowledge that he was seeking. He was a very famous person and was used to taking charge of his affairs. However, we were in my territory and I would be of no benefit if I allowed him to do whatever he wanted. Maybe that's why doctors have big desks and place people in small chairs or funny gowns. It always gives us the upper hand. I am not saying that doctors need to be superior, just on an equal footing. That is the beauty of a doctor's office. Everyone is equal. No one is more important or can escape any disease because of money or prestige or power. It is like being in church or synagogue - it doesn't matter what one has accomplished or how much money one has, G-d will look at you as the type of person you are and how you have acted to others.

Mr. Wilkens was upset about having to take so many pills. He said that they didn't make him feel well and made him fatigued. He needed more energy in order to work. He said that he was mainly sedentary and painted all day long, in his studio. He very rarely went outdoors anymore. He painted from memory or from photos. When he did sculptures, he worked in the studio as well. He did not do them too much anymore, because he found it fatiguing. On further interrogation, he said that when he walked for a short period, he would get short of breath. He also complained of pain his calves when he walked. If he would stop walking the shortness of breath and the calf pain would go away. He had complained of having to wake up in the night to urinate at least 4-5 times per night. He said in his gruff manner " getting up to piss every hour makes me tired all day long. I can't get a good night's sleep anymore." He also complained about his inability to walk and get exercise, " how I am supposed to lose weight, when I can't even walk? I get short of breath and my damn legs start to hurt so much that I can't exercise at all." He was very angry. I wondered if his anger was reflected in his paintings - I never saw an angry deer.

I told him "let's try to do things in an orderly manner." Let's review your previous records, go over your medications, do a complete exam, and then we can discuss what we need to do to try and get you to feel better". He seemed to calm down when I put everything in order. At least I didn't just push him out and tell him to come back when he lost weight. It's too easy to blame everything on obesity or eating too much. The patient sometimes doesn't have control over their weight gain - it just happens. His work was very important to him and he couldn't get out into the woods to view the wildlife. His work and personal life were suffering due to his inability to walk. He had bad leg pain and would get very short of breath with minimal exertion. Obviously, something wasn't right and the situation already sounded very dangerous for his health.

He was on about 5 medications for control of his blood pressure - he had severe Hypertension (high blood pressure) and diabetes. Some of the medications were adversely interacting with others. Many of the bottles of pills had different doctors' names on them. He told me he was dissatisfied with his doctors and kept looking for new ones. I thought that not all of the doctors he saw knew exactly which medications he was taking. After reviewing his medications, I read the medical records that he brought with him to the office. He only had a few notes from several doctors. The records were mainly about adjusting his medications and trying to get him to lose weight and get his blood pressure down. Everybody was completely unsuccessful on all accounts.

I then began my exam of Mr. Wilkens. His body mass index (BMI) was very high at 38. Anything over 30 is considered obese. His blood pressure was 178/103 - very high, and this was despite being on several medications to lower the pressure. This was very dangerous as such a high blood pressure can precipitate a stroke or heart attack or cause kidney failure. I first examined his eyes with a special scope - an ophthalmoscope. This revealed changes in the eye due to uncontrolled high blood pressure. Usually if the blood vessels in the eye have been affected by hypertension, then, other vessels in the body are also damaged. This is a sign that his blood pressure has been out of control for an extended period of time.

I then examined his neck and listened to the carotid arteries with my stethoscope. I heard bruits. This means that the arteries in the neck, that feed the brain with blood, have been narrowed. This is a very ominous sign and requires further attention. The remained of his exam including the heart exam and the lungs were normal. Mr. Wilkens had an enormous abdomen and his belly hung over the front of his pants. It looked like his abdomen had become bigger lately, because his pants were so tight on him. He was not a smoker and that probably saved his life. If he had been a smoker, surely a major stroke or heart attack would have occurred by now. His legs exam revealed that he had decreased pulses to his feet. This was why he was having pain in his legs when he walked. The blood vessels that fed his lower extremities with blood and thus oxygen were blocked. This was most likely from plaques of cholesterol blocking the arteries of the legs (see figures 12-a, 12-b).

We then did some lab studies on his blood and urine. This revealed that he had diabetes with a blood sugar of 300. He also had mild kidney failure. There was protein in the urine, which told me that his kidneys weren't working well. He probably had uncontrolled high blood pressure and diabetes for a while. His other lab studies were abnormal as well. He had very high cholesterol and very high triglycerides (another fat in the bloodstream). His LDL (the bad cholesterol - the one that deposits cholesterol in the arteries) was elevated. His HDL (the good cholesterol - the one that removes the cholesterol form the arteries) was too low.

I spoke with Mr. Wilkens and his wife. She was very concerned about him. She stated that he hadn't looked well for a while. He was getting up a lot during the night to urinate and he wasn't sleeping well. He would become short of breath with walking. He had severe pain in his legs with walking a short distance. " What is wrong with him?" she pleaded. " We went to several doctors and they all told us he needs to lose weight. I am so concerned about my husband." She went on to tell me that he had a display of his work in a museum and he didn't go, because he wasn't feeling well. She felt that bringing him to Florida would help, but it didn't. His symptoms began to progress and he became worse.

"He has **Syndrome X**", I said. "What the hell is that" he responded." "Sit down, calm down and let's go over the whole thing. I have some free time and we can talk about what you have and what we need to do." I began to explain, "Syndrome X is also called, **Metabolic Syndrome.** It is a new name that we assign to patients with certain problems, like you have. It includes, being overweight and having high blood sugar. The other characteristics of Syndrome X are having a lot of abdominal fat, high blood pressure, and plaque buildup in the arteries."

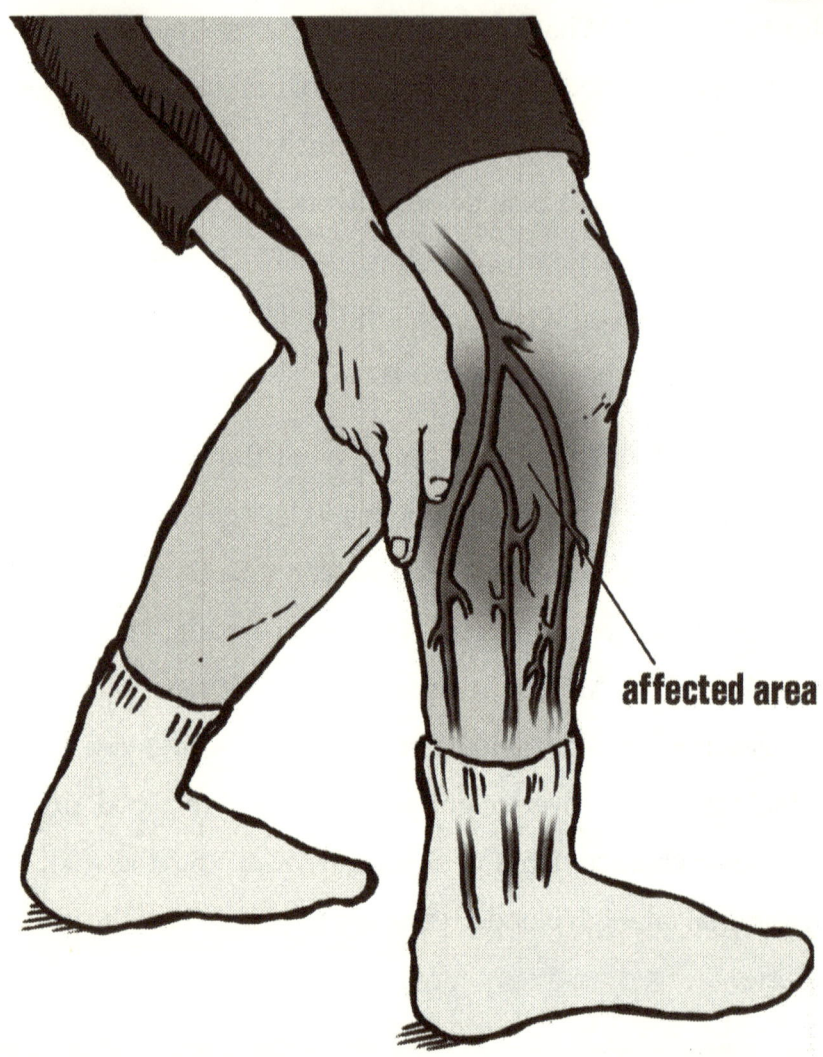

affected area

Fig. 12-a. Peripheral vascular disease - the patient gets pain in the legs while walking. Then, the pain will go away with rest. This is called claudication. This is due to an occlusion or blockage of the arteries of the legs.

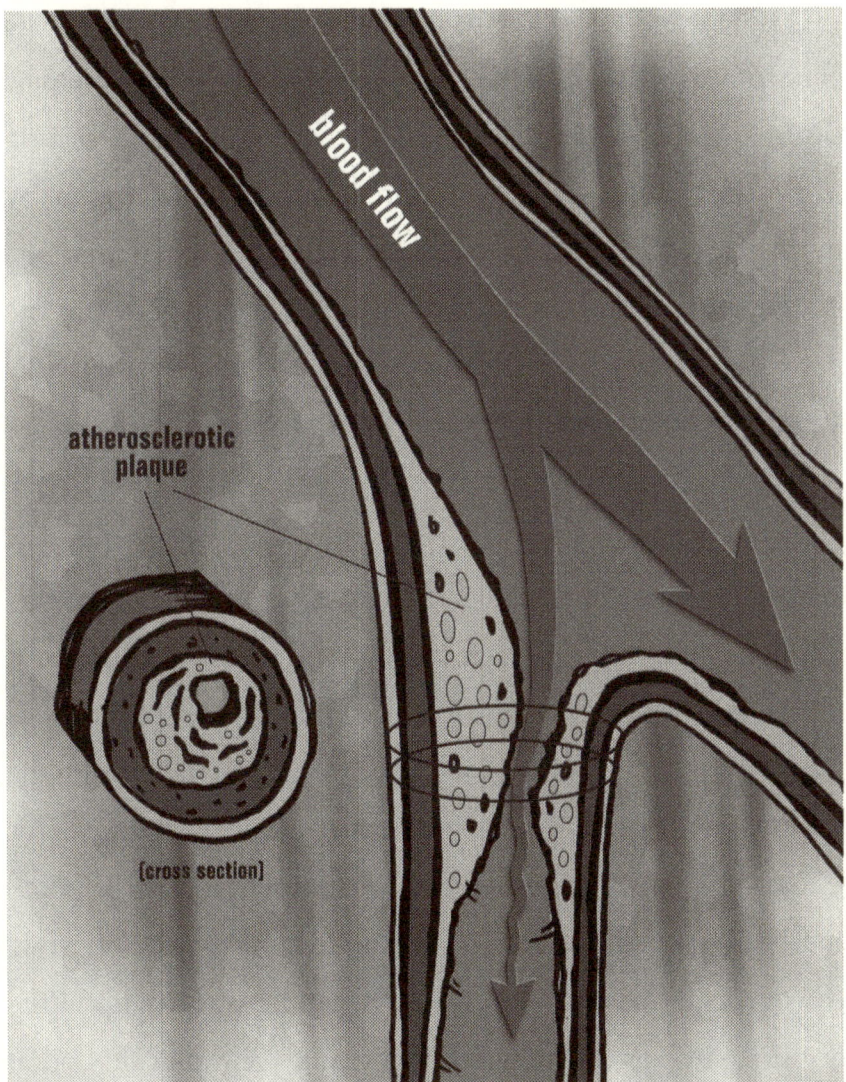

Fig. 12-b. Occluded artery of the leg. The flow of blood through the artery is blocked. This causes pain in the area that doesn't get enough blood.

I proceeded to explain as best and simply as I could, "The syndrome is a disease of the body's metabolism. When someone starts to put on weight, the body has difficulty metabolizing sugar. Normally, sugar is lowered in the bloodstream by insulin. This comes from the pancreas, an organ that sits in the back of the abdomen. When the sugar goes up, the pancreas secretes more insulin. In patients with the metabolic syndrome, the insulin doesn't work. For some reason the high body fat creates a situation of **insulin resistance**. So the body keeps more sugar in the bloodstream. The pancreas keeps secreting more and more insulin - which is a storage hormone. This causes even more fat deposition. Ultimately, the pancreas burns out and no more insulin is secreted. This leads to an even higher blood sugar and diabetes. For some reason, people with this disorder can't use insulin efficiently. Thus, your ability to process sugar is impaired. At this point, the body has diabetes and metabolic syndrome. The body can't process the fats, like cholesterol and they buildup in the arteries, such as in the heart and brain. We are at this point with Mr. Wilkens" I said. " I believe that he has many arteries blocked by the plaques of cholesterol and clots. His kidneys have been damaged by the diabetes and high blood pressure and he is in imminent danger of having a heart attack and a stroke". Mrs. Wilkens asked " is this disease common, I never heard of it?" I told her " it has been estimated that over 50 million Americans have this problem. It will continue to get worse as the incidence of obesity rises. It has not received a lot of attention in the media - but it will."

She asked me, "what do we do now?" I answered, "since his disease is so far along, let's place him in the hospital and run a few tests. I don't think it would be safe to treat this as an outpatient at this time. He is in too much danger." I think that Mr. And Mrs. Wilkens were relieved. Finally, they were getting some answers about what was wrong with him. Mr. Wilkens can be very overpowering and previously wouldn't follow the doctor's orders. Now, he is feeling so bad and his work and life have been suffering He was willing to do anything at this time to feel better. I also believe that he was now scared and would submit to a more comprehensive medical evaluation.

Mr. Wilkens was admitted to the hospital. I adjusted his medications to control his high blood pressure. He was placed on insulin therapy to bring down his blood sugar (glucose). He was placed on blood thinners to prevent a stroke. A cardiologist saw him in consultation and a cardiac catheterization was recommended. This is an angiogram of the coronary arteries, to determine how much blockage there is in the arteries around the heart (fig. 12-c). He also had a Doppler study, that is, a non-invasive study of his arteries in the legs and neck. Mr. Wilkens remained compliant through his tests.

He didn't like having them done. He was a man that was used to being in charge. Here, he was just another patient. Being a patient made him feel out of control and weak. However, he knew these tests were necessary and he would not get better without them. He was very anxious to get back to his work and start painting again. He would put up with anything to feel good again.

Mr. Wilkens started feeling better right away. With his blood sugar and blood pressure under control, he was not as hostile and became friendlier. He told me that he was feeling better and having less mood swings. We placed him on a low-fat, diabetic diet (table 12-a, at the end of this chapter) and he was initially having trouble eating this. He felt hungry at first and then after a few days, he became used to it. I sat down with him and his wife to review all of the test results. We were in his patient room and he was walking around with an IV attached to a pole. He was receiving IV fluids to keep his kidneys working. This is frequently done after a catheterization to wash out the dye used in the procedure.

I started speaking with his chart in my hands. I said, "let's go over the heart catheterization first, okay?" He replied "sure thing." The heart catheterization revealed 2 major blockages in his coronary arteries (Fig. 12-c). In fact, I told him " you were ready to have a heart attack at any moment." I saw on his chart that the cardiologist had already scheduled him for an angioplasty the next morning. His arteries in the neck (the carotid arteries) were also occluded, but should be able to be managed medically. That means without surgical intervention. The legs arteries were another story. They were almost completely occluded, and he would require a surgical procedure at a later date. Of course, the heart procedure would come first.

He underwent the angioplasty the next morning. This was done by one of the cardiologists. The cardiologist was able to open up the two blocked arteries with a balloon. He then inserted a stent to keep the arteries open (fig.12-d). The procedure was uneventful and we talked about hospital discharge. If the artery could not be opened or the stents could not be placed, then he would have required a bypass surgery. This is an operation where the occlusion in an artery is bypasses using either the patients own veins or arteries (fig.12-e).

Prior to leaving the hospital, he was seen by a dietician and a nutritionist. He will need to lose weight and be on a special diet for the remainder of his life. He will be on insulin for a while, to keep his blood glucose down. He asked me " will I have to stay on insulin forever?" I answered " no, not necessarily. If you lose weight, then you may be able to get by with just being on pills to lower the blood sugar. In fact, I have had several patients like you, that have been able to come off of all of their medications, with weight loss and proper diets." He was happy with that and seemed determined to get his life back and to take control of his eating habits. He will have to give up his sugary sodas. " I used to drink 10 cans of coke a day," he said. I told him that a can of soda has about 20 teaspoons of sugar in it and it uses, HFCS (high fructose - corn syrup). This can cause rapid weight gain and insulin release. Just by giving that up, you will feel much better. He asked me how to get the weight off, and I replied, "that is a very slow process. You may be a candidate for a gastric bypass if dieting and exercise don't work. However, I believe that you will do well with the dieting."

He was able to go home the next morning. He will have to come back in a few weeks for his surgery to bypass the arteries in his legs. That is a major procedure and I am hoping that there won't be any problems with that. He went home on several medications. He was on 1 Aspirin a day and Plavix 1 per day. These are blood thinners that prevents clots from forming in the arteries. They will help maintain the arteries patent. He is on insulin and I placed him on Lantus insulin - this is just one shot every night and is very easy to administer. He is on an ARB, (Angiotensin Receptor Blocker) to control his blood pressure. He has already lost 5 pounds in a short hospital stay, had his arteries to his heart opened and a stent placed. His blood pressure was controlled with medications. His blood sugar was stabilized on one little dose of insulin at night as well as the diet. I made him an appointment to come to my office in a few days.

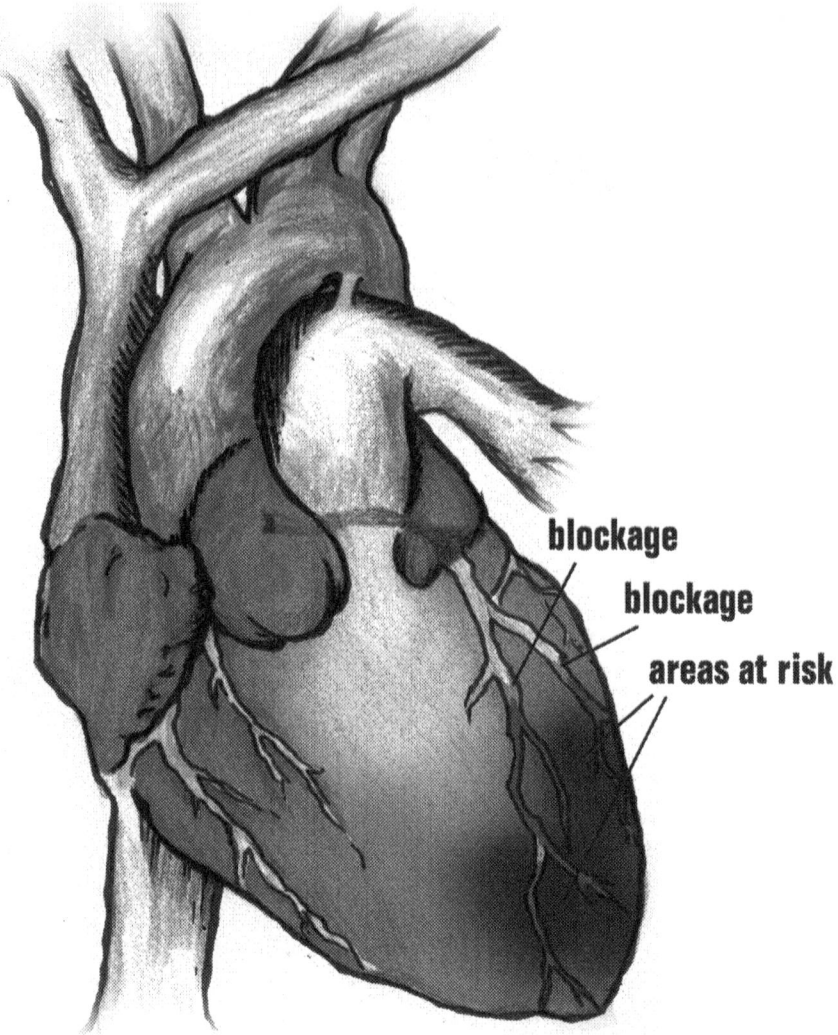

Fig. 12-c. The heart catheterization reveals two blockages. Blood can't flow very well past the blockages. Thus, no oxygen can get to the tissues past the blockages. This can lead to death of the heart tissue (heart attack).

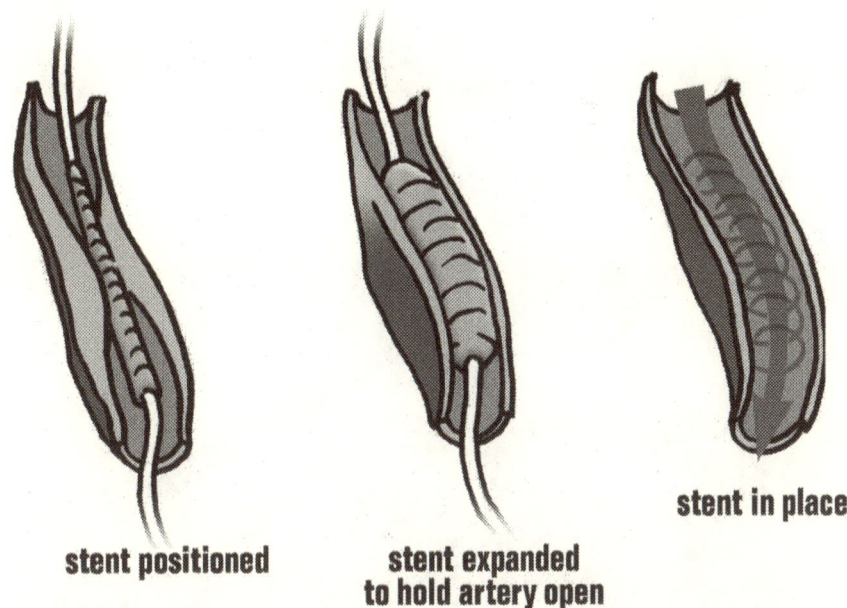

stent positioned   **stent expanded**   **stent in place**
                           to hold artery open

Fig. 12-d. This is how the stent is placed. A catheter is passed into the coronary artery and an angioplasty is performed. The stent is then inserted and stays in the artery. The stent is like a little cage that helps to keep the artery open. The stent remains in the artery after the procedure is finished, to help keep the artery open.

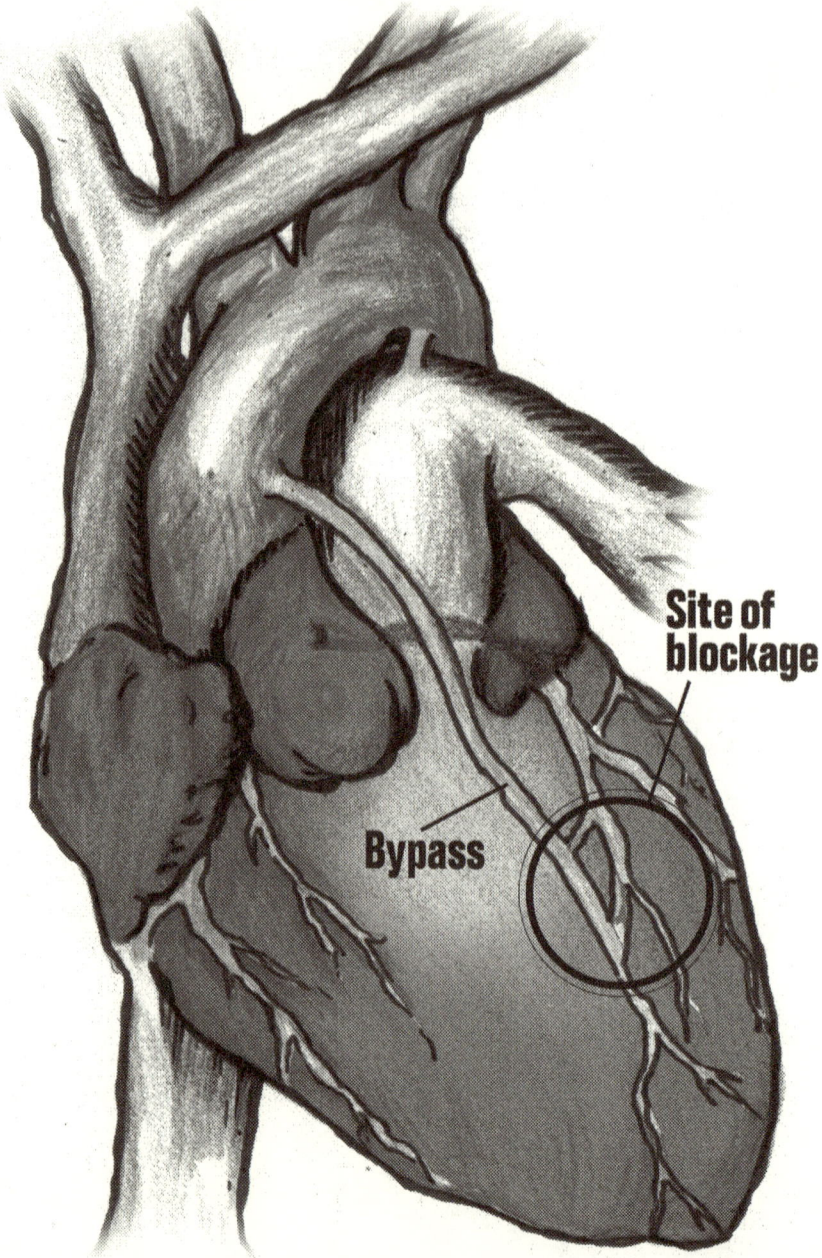

Fig. 12-e. This is a heart where one artery has been bypassed. This shows the artery on the right side of the heart with a bypass graft.

He came back with his wife for the next office visit. He was a much nicer man than on his previous exam. His wife and I agreed that the elevated blood glucose and high blood pressure were causing him to have some personality changes. A high blood sugar can actually cause some swelling of the brain and subsequent personality changes. He looked much better. He had more color in his face and he said that the shortness of breath had been much reduced. He said that the pain in his legs was also better and he wanted to reconsider whether he wanted to have that surgery. He wanted to see if there would be some disease regression on diet and medications. I checked his cholesterol in the office and it had improved, but was still elevated. I added a statin to his medical regimen. He was placed on Crestor, one tablet daily. This should help lower his bad cholesterol and triglycerides and raise his HDL (the good cholesterol). In addition, it may help prevent re-occlusion of his coronary arteries. Crestor and other statins (Zocor, Lipitor, Pravachol, etc.) can even promote regression of the cholesterol plaques in his carotids and the arteries of his legs.

After the office visit, he walked to his car and re-entered the office. He was carrying a box or something under a huge sheet. He said that he had something for me. I pulled off the drape and there was a very large painting of a mountain lion. He said, "this was going to be placed in a show, but I want you to have it instead. I really appreciated your care and personal attention that you have given to me. I was taken aback and shocked. I knew how much effort went into his making a picture like that. I also realized that is was something very valuable and told him so. He said," this is not nearly as valuable as my life and this is from my wife and I." This was a very touching gesture and I really appreciated it and told him so. It is now in the lobby of my office and when I see it think of the mountain lion that had been tamed into a house cat. All it took was some patience and good medical care.

Truth and Reality

The metabolic syndrome is a well - documented disease that will increase in notoriety in the near future. It is caused by insulin resistance - that is, resistance to a hormone that is responsible for regulating the sugar in your body. It is associated with obesity. People in America are becoming more obese and it is even starting in children and young adults. The clinical problems associated with the metabolic syndrome are central obesity, blood fat disorders, and blockages in arteries, diabetes, and an elevated cholesterol level. The syndrome is caused by obesity and the disease can make the obesity even worse. The treatment is weight loss, diet control and exercise. For someone with this disease, weight loss and proper medical care is mandatory. If the patient cannot lose weight on their own, then diet pills or a gastric bypass should be considered.

The number of people with this syndrome in the USA is estimated to be over 50 million. Thus, we can see the enormity of this problem. Obesity is a major health hazard. Persons with a BMI over 30 should routinely have their blood glucose, lipoproteins (cholesterol and LDL and HDL), and blood pressure checked. The arteries of patients with metabolic syndrome should also be checked with Doppler studies. Pain in the legs while walking can be a sign of occluded arteries of the legs. The heart should be evaluated with a stress test or nuclear studies. Inflammation in the body may be increased in patients with the metabolic syndrome. This can be checked with a blood test called a C-reactive Protein (CRP).

Patients with the metabolic syndrome should be placed on a very aggressive weight loss program. A dietician should monitor them. If necessary, diet medications may be used to assist with the weight loss. There are a lot of new diet drugs on the horizon and many of them look promising. Gastric bypass is another alternative, if weight loss is unsuccessful with diet and exercise. I am hopeful that new gastric procedures will be developed for weight reduction. The gastric stimulator looks very promising and I hope that it will be introduced into the USA very soon.

If a doctor tells you that you have the metabolic syndrome or syndrome X, you should follow their instructions very carefully. It is important to follow their weight loss and exercise programs. Avoid sugar and fatty foods. Limit your caloric intake to less than 2,000 calories per day and maybe even less. Avoid foods with HFCS, as this can increase the insulin release. The blood pressure can become very elevated and you must take your medications on a regular basis. Make daily exercise a part of your life. It will help you look younger and live longer.

Table 12-a. **The Diabetic Diet (Low -fat)**

This is a healthy low-fat, diabetic diet. This will provide from 1500-1800 calories per day. This diet can be followed by anyone that wishes to be on a healthy low-sugar, low-fat diet.

Breakfast:

English muffin, toast, a bagel with margarine or ½ cup of a cereal with milk (skim).
Banana or strawberries or any fruit that you desire.
Cocoa mix (artificially sweetened), coffee or tea.

Lunch:

Tortilla with chicken or a turkey sandwich on bread of choice and mustard
or low-fat mayonnaise, with lettuce and tomato
Vegetable of choice - corn, beans, carrots or any other vegetable.
You may have a small salad with a low-fat dressing
Juice - low-sugar or a diet soda
Fruit or a yogurt for dessert

Dinner:

Chicken - 2 oz., hamburger or a steak (lean meats), fish - tuna steak or another low-fat fish, turkey - white meat. You may have ½ cup of cooked pasta with a low-fat sauce
Peas or another vegetable, 3 oz. Potato - baked
Salad - low-fat dressing
Fruit for dessert

Evening snack:

Low-fat milk, popcorn, non-sweetened ices, yogurt, or fruit

Seasonings that may be added:

Flavoring extracts
Garlic - fresh or powder
Herbs
Mustard
Soy Sauce
Red wine vinegar

13 | Obtaining Health Insurance

Health is not valued, until sickness comes."
Dr. Thomas Fuller (1654-1734)

Health insurance is the most important insurance that you must have. What can possibly be more crucial than to have access to proper health care? You need to have health insurance to ensure that in a time of need, you and your family will get the best of care. Not having health insurance can be devastating to both your health and your financial well-being.

The most important step in obtaining proper medical care is signing up with the right health insurance plan. It is crucial to find the plan that will be correct for your needs. Since most insurance plans are provided through employment, your choices may be limited. It is so important to review the policies of the different plans being offered to you. The time to do this is <u>not</u> when you are ill. The time to review the policies is when you are being offered the plans at work. Unfortunately, most people will spend less time reviewing the health plans than they will in deciding what type of topping should go on their pizza for dinner. The average person will get the policy, stuff it into a drawer, and hope they never have to look at it again. That is understandable, since the plans can be so complex. Let me try to highlight the most salient features for you to consider, when choosing a plan.

Choosing the right plan for you and your family should be done at the time of enrollment into the plan. You have to look at the **benefits** of the plan. There are so many questions that you have to think of. The most crucial one: What is covered? In other words, does this plan pay for doctors and hospitals, tests, X-rays, etc. How much are the **deductible and co-pays**? You may be able to select a plan that has larger deductibles and co-pays and then less may be taken out of the paycheck. That brings us to how much does it cost? Obviously, most people want the most coverage for the least amount of money.

Most employers will pay a part of the insurance premium. The remainder of the premium is left for the employee to pay. The employee's part will be taken out of the paycheck, so it's important to know how much the employer will share in paying for the premium. If you very rarely have to go to the doctor, you want a plan with larger co-pays and deductibles. On the other hand, if you have a chronic illness (such as diabetes), and have to go to the doctor frequently, select a plan with lower co-pays. This will be more cost-effective.

There are many other factors to consider when selecting a health plan:

Does the plan have a prescription benefit? If there is a prescription benefit, will it cover brand names as well as generic? Are the medications that you are taking, covered as a tier 1 (reduced prescription co-pay)? Will your insurance cover Injectibles? Medicines such as Epogen, Ribavirins, anti-arthritic medications, are now routinely used, and can cost thousands of dollars a month. If you are taking or may need such medications, make certain that the plan you choose will pay for these medications. A little homework up front can potentially save you thousands of dollars.

How well does the insurance plan cover your dependents? Is there a different co-pay and deductible for your family? You need to know how much of the monthly premium you are responsible for and how much is paid by the employer. Find out if the coverage includes your children and their immunizations. You need to know if the insurance will cover your children if they are in college, and after they leave home. Does the insurance cover your children if they live away from home? It may be cheaper to buy insurance from a college or university than to have regular commercial insurance.

There are many items in the insurance policy that you need to know. It is imperative that you find out what you will be responsible for **prior to an illness**. You don't want to come home from the hospital, after a major surgery, to find out that your insurance carrier didn't cover this illness or the doctor or hospital. You don't want to hold your breath while opening the hospital invoice. Find out how much is the **out of pocket limit**. This means how much you have to pay before the insurance carrier will pick up at 100%. You should ask the agent what is the "worst case scenario". In other words, at what point of a major hospitalization or illness, does the carrier start paying it entirely. A better insurance will limit your "out of pocket " expense. You also need to know if your carrier can cut off your benefits in the middle of an illness. In the unfortunate possibility that you or a dependent gets a major illness (i.e. AIDS, Leukemia, Hepatitis C), can the carrier terminate your coverage in the middle of treatment and leave you stranded.

Find out if your policy has benefits for Ophthalmology or Dental care. If everybody in your family wears glasses or have poor dentition, you will want this type of insurance. Will it kick in for braces (Orthodontics)? I had braces put on my children, it cost many thousands of dollars, and I had no coverage for this. However, when my children smile at me, I know that it was worth every penny.

Another important item is substance abuse. Does your carrier pay for a rehabilitation facility for drug and alcohol abuse? This type of treatment can easily run into the many tens of thousands of dollars. Most carriers will have a limited benefit for the treatment of substance abuse. The average stay in a rehabilitation facility is three months with costs of about $ 15,000 - $20,000 per month. This can humble most people's savings. The last thing an alcoholic or drug user needs is no insurance for their treatment. And make certain that the carrier will pay for treatment in a good facility. You don't want to place a family member in a poor quality treatment center. They can come out worse than they went in. Find out if the rehabilitation coverage is only for certain centers that give the insurance carrier a discount. This means that the rehab facility is not highly regarded and may not provide the best chance at recovery.

When signing up for a particular plan, you need to look at the doctor list. Find out which doctors and hospitals are participating in this plan. Look at the doctor list and see if your Physician is on that list. You don't want to change doctors due to the plan. If your doctor is not on the list, the plan is most likely not paying the doctors enough money. Some plans will try to cut down on their overhead by scrimping on the amount that they pay the Physicians. You don't want an unhappy Physician providing your medical care. The payment to Physicians is usually based on the Medicare reimbursement. The truth is that most plans exactly copy the amount of money they pay to doctors from Medicare. Some plans will give slightly more. The lower quality plans will usually give less. The Physicians are usually unable to discuss the amount of reimbursement to the patients, as part of a confidentially agreement with the plan. What can you do? When signing up for the plan, find out how the doctors are being reimbursed for their services. The last thing you need is a doctor that is being paid less than the standard, for services rendered. You don't want to be in the economy section when you could have been in first class. The above has been written for patients who have access to coverage through an employer. What about health coverage for those who are self-employed or are between jobs? For these people, I would strongly advise to go on the Internet and look for a Website that will provide you with health insurance plans. A good place to start is **www.ehealthinsurance.com.** This can give you different quotes from different insurance carriers. When you see the quotes and find one for you, then you can go ahead and fill out the detailed applications. Also, other websites such as **www.insurance.com,** which will give you several different health insurance plans by different companies. You can try and adjust your plan for the type of premium that you want to pay, as well as if you have pre-existing illnesses, etc. If you are uninsurable due to a serious illness, pre-existing claims, then you can look at some state programs, which run things known as "risk pools". The Website for this is **www.naschip.org/states**. This will give you links to certain state programs. The different premiums that you may wish to consider will depend on how frequently you will need the health insurance, certain underlying illnesses and whether you have young children and wish to have them under your plan or not. Certainly if you get health insurance through a group or through your employer, that would be the best option, but that may not be available for everybody.

What about if you have **Medicare** as your primary insurance? Most people over the age of 65 have Medicare. Should you get a secondary policy? The answer is an unequivocal yes! It is important to have a secondary policy that will cover the 20% of the costs that Medicare doesn't pay for. A good secondary insurance will also pay for your Medicare deductible that is now $110 per calendar year. In addition, a good secondary policy to Medicare will be an **automatic crossover**. That means that it will pay the 20% that Medicare doesn't pay without the claims coming to you. The claims from the Doctor or hospital will go directly from Medicare to the secondary insurance carrier. You won't have to be bothered by filing the secondary insurance yourself.

Should you join an HMO and give up your Medicare policy? That depends on your financial status and your health. If you like to travel and are financially independent, keep your regular Medicare with a supplemental policy. If you are on a lot of medicines and an HMO will pay for them, you may wish to go with an HMO - Medicare. However, the HMO will restrict which Doctors and hospitals you can go to. The HMO may also prevent you from having certain testing and only provide you with generic medications. In choosing whether to assign your benefits to an HMO - you must consider that an HMO will impose many restrictions on your care. However, an HMO will be less expensive for you, especially if you require a lot of medical care and take multiple, expensive medications.

Should you consider a **health savings account** (HSA)? This is a savings account that acts like an IRA. The money goes into this account and is used for medical expenses. If you don't use this money, you usually get to keep it, tax-free. This type of account is usually paired with a high-deductible health care policy. When the deductible needs to be met, the money is taken from the savings account. The money in the savings account will be used for the deductible and any other medical costs i.e. medications and co-pays. This type of policy, the HSA, will gain in popularity in the future. It is a means to attempt to reduce the costs of medical care and health insurance.

Truth and Reality

There are two ways that Physicians are paid by insurance carriers. Why should you care? Because it will impact your health care. Physicians are either "**capitated** " or paid a "**fee-for-service**". Capitated means that the Physician has a list of patients and he gets a small amount of money per patient per month. The more patients on the list, the more money. It doesn't matter if the doctor sees the patient or not - the Physician is paid the same. In a fee-for-service system, the doctor will bill the insurance carrier each time the patient is seen, whether in the office or hospital. In this type of plan, the doctor gets paid only when a patient is examined and treated. Thus, in a capitated plan the Physician will make money whether the patient is seen or never goes to the doctor. In a fee-for- service plan, the doctor is paid only when the patient goes to the office. Stay away from capitated plans! Physicians don't like them and it is not a good business.

When you look at the Physician list, check to see if the Physician that you wish to go to is Board Certified. There will be a star next to the Physician's name in the doctor and hospital roster. A star next to the Physician's name will indicate that he has completed all of the training to be a specialist in their particular field. It also tells you that the doctor has passed his specialty boards. This means that the doctor has worked very hard and is more likely to be a higher quality Physician than one that has not passed their boards.

Make certain that the hospital of your choice is a **participating provider** with your insurance plan. This will mean that there will not be extra fees for you to pay, if you want to go to your usual hospital. Sometimes, an insurance company will contract with a lesser quality hospital to save money. You may be excluded from going to the hospital of your choice. It may be necessary for you to have to go to a hospital far from home to be covered under your insurance plan. So, make certain that the hospital of your choice is a participating provider with your prospective insurance carrier.

Another factor for you to consider when signing up for an insurance plan, is if the plan is **medically underwritten**. This means that you can be excluded from the plan if you are very sick. Are there **pre-existing conditions** that your plan will not pay for? Don't think that you can fool your plan. If you don't give them all of the correct information when you sign up, they can refuse to pay for any claims that you incur at a later date. The insurance carriers are very smart and know all of the tricks. They will obtain all of your medical records to see if they can refuse to pay any claims. Make certain that you will not have any pre-existing exclusions to your medical coverage. If you have a chronic illness, let your insurance carrier know up front and make sure that they will cover you if this illness gets worse.

You also need to know whether your insurance is an individual or a group policy. An individual policy can be kept forever (although with increasing premiums as you age). A group policy can be terminated at any time. This last type of policy can have increasing rates on a class basis and not on personal claims. A group policy can be terminated at any time and can have the premiums increased based on your group's utilization of services. In other words, if your group (employer and co-employees) causes the carrier to lose money, they will raise your rates. An individual policy may cost more, but it can't be terminated as a group policy can.

Make certain that you have heard of the carrier and that it has a good reputation. You can look up the carrier on the Internet to make certain that it is solvent. Do not waste your premiums on a fly-by-night carrier. They are known in the business as street policies or "Podunk Mutual". They will not be there when you need them, that is, when you have claims to be paid.

The purchasing of health insurance can be a daunting task. If your employer allows you to have options for different policies, educate yourself and review the policies. Having the right policy can insure that you and your family get the healthcare that you need and deserve. It can also save you a significant sum of money by having the right policy in place at the right time.

Summary: when choosing an insurance plan, find out:

- How much **coverage** you will receive.
- Amount of **deductible and co-pays.**
- Amount of **maternity** and can you add or delete this coverage as per your needs.
- **Medication co-pays** and eligibility for **brand names** and **Injectibles**
- What is the **out-of-pocket limit** and worst-case scenario?

? Is there coverage for **substance abuse and mental health** and what are the limits on this coverage? Is there a restriction on rehabilitation facilities?

? Are your **favorite doctors and hospitals** providers on this insurance coverage?

? Is the policy **medically underwritten** and will you be excluded for a **pre-existing** illness?

? Does the carrier have a **good reputation** and are they financially solvent?

Good luck in getting the best medical insurance. I placed this almost last in this book, but it may be the most important step in staying healthy.

14 | Making a Doctor's Appointment

"Art of medicine consists in amusing the patient while nature cures the disease."
Voltaire (1694 - 1778)

Most people find a doctor by word-of-mouth. That is, they will ask a relative or friend whom they like as a Physician and then see that doctor. However, the situation is much more complex at this time. You need to be certain that the Physician that you want to see is a provider for your insurance plan. Even more important, will this doctor and their staff meet your needs?

If you are in search of a new Physician, the time to start looking is when you are feeling well. It is imperative that you become established with a new Physician, before an illness. If you are ill, the Physician may not be able to take on a new patient, at that time. The last thing you want is to have to go to an Emergency Room (ER) when you are ill. The wait may be very long and the quality of the Physicians may not be what you need. In addition, your co-pay will be much higher and the claims from the ER may not be covered by your insurance plan. Sometimes, an insurance carrier will deny claims from an ER, if a Physicians office could provide the services. The reason for this is simple - the ER bill may be up to 10 times more than an office visit. You may end up being responsible for the ER bills - ouch!

The first step in selecting your Physician is to go to the directory of Physicians provided by your insurance carrier. Look in either primary care or under a particular specialty that you need. Most of the time, you cannot go directly to a specialist. You may need a referral from the Primary Care Physician (PCP). Look in the directory under primary care, family physicians, or internal medicine. If you are an adult and don't want children in the examining rooms and lobby, then select internal medicine. If you want a doctor to take care of you and your children, you may prefer a family physician. I limit my practice to 17 years of age and older. I love children, but I don't like to hear them cry and scream, while I am at work.

Select several possible candidates that you would consider to be your Physician. You may recognize some of the names and they may have excellent reputations. This may make your search easier. Of course, the location of the office is important. Select one that is either near your home or work, for your convenience. Make certain that the Physician that you select is on staff at the hospital that you prefer. Only select Physicians that are Board-Certified in their specialty (a star next to their name). This will guarantee you that your Physician has completed their medical training and is a leader in their field. It will be hard to tell if you have selected a good Physician by their names alone. Certainly, most people will select a male or female based on their preference. In addition, if you require another language to be spoken, that should be in the directory. If the Physician is accepting new patients, that will be listed in the directory, along with office hours. Make certain that the doctor's schedule will meet yours. If you are working full time, see if the doctor has evening or weekend hours.

The next step in selecting the Physician is to call the office. This is a crucial step. You want to be able to contact the office and make an appointment. If the phone is not answered or someone picks up and says, "hold please", these are very bad signs. If you get a voice mail or a machine, leave a message and see how long it takes to get back to you. If you are placed to an answering service, that is not bad. At least you get to speak to somebody and they can give you instructions. Always get the name of the person you speak with. Of course, it would be best if you can get directly through to the office and speak with the doctor's staff.

If you can't get through to the doctor's office, you may wish to select another Physician. How can you develop a relationship with a Physician, if you can't even get in to see them? From the doctor's standpoint, hiring personnel to answer phones is expensive. They may be busy enough and not care if people can get through to the office on a timely basis. The insurance companies have reduced the Physician reimbursement down so much that the doctor cannot afford to hire front office personnel. The doctor has to do so many things to keep the office going and answering the phones may not be high on the list. However, your <u>only</u> concern is getting high quality healthcare. The problems that the doctors encounter are simply not an issue for you to be concerned with. In the future, it will be even more difficult to negotiate the web of managed care and this will require more skill on your part.

Once you find an office that has the proper phone skills and personnel, you need to set up an appointment. You should discuss the following issues with the telephone receptionist: Is the appointment at your **desired time**? What are the **office's hours**? What is the **average waiting time** to get in for an illness? **How long is the wait** in the waiting room (that's why it's called a waiting room, silly)? Will you be **seeing the Physician you're requested or another Physician or a Physician's Assistant**? **What will be done** on the first visit? Will I have a **complete exam?** What clothes should I **wear?** Sometimes you need loose fitting and no tight sleeves, etc. Can you get my **previous medical records and laboratory studies** there for the visit or do I need to bring them? Very important!! This will help the Physician a great deal and it will make you a more important and intelligent consumer of healthcare. Will the doctor be ordering laboratory studies and will they be done on the premises? Confirm that this Physician is a provider for your insurance carrier and this hasn't changed. Will there be **paperwork to be completed?** If so, you may wish to go to the office and complete them prior to your visit. This will also give you the opportunity to see and **inspect the office,** prior to the actual office visit.

Truth and Reality

A Physician that is interested in doing a good job and providing excellent medical care, will take care of the business part of the practice. If the phone is answered promptly and courteously, more than likely, you will be satisfied with the medical care. If the phone is not answered, or the staff is rude and hostile - stay away! If the exam rooms are neat and clean and the staff looks professional, these are good signs that you will be happy and that the practice is well run. Make sure that you only go to a practice where the Physician is being paid for a fee-for-service and is not capitated. You don't want to be "herded" through and receive a poor quality service. Remember that you are really paying the doctor and not the insurance carrier. Money is being taken out of your paycheck for these services and you should expect and demand high - quality medical care.

Summary

• Find a Physician as soon as you receive the medical coverage - do _not_ wait until you are ill to establish yourself with a doctor.

• Make certain that your new Physician is **Board-Certified**.

• Find a doctor that will be **close to your home or work**. You may need to find a doctor with evening or weekend hours to fit your schedule.

• Get your **previous medical records to the new doctor before your visit** or bring them with you.

Complete all of the paperwork before your visit. Ask the receptionist to mail them to you at the time of the scheduling of your first visit.

Make certain that the Physician you select is on **active staff at your preferred hospital**.

Call the new Physicians office and see "how it feels". Is the staff friendly and courteous? Are the phones answered promptly and is there an after hour answering service?

Visit the office and determine if it will meet your needs. Is the **office clean and professional**?

Does the Physician employ Physician - extenders i.e. **nurse practitioners and Physician Assistants?** If there are Physician extenders, that means the doctor is busy and has available help. This will make it easier for you to be seen.

Make certain that the doctor is being reimbursed on a "**fee-for -service**" basis.

15 | The First Office Visit

The first visit to your new Physician's office is very important to obtaining proper health care. It is the time for you to decide whether to proceed with this Physician or to look elsewhere for health care. You need to come prepared for this visit! Not only do you need to bring the proper documents, but also you need to come armed with a sharp eye and mind.

You have to decide if the office is in the right location for you. Make certain that the drive to the office is not too far from your home or place of employment. In the event that you can't have a car, make sure that there is public transportation for you to use. Don't forget that you may be coming here a lot and you want the location to be convenient.

When you pull up in your car, take a look around. You can ask yourself:

Is the office professional looking, clean, with brightly colored signage? Is it safe or is it next to a bar with unsavory characters lurking around? Is the parking adequate and are there spaces close to the office? Is it wheelchair accessible and are there designated parking spaces for the disabled? Go with your gut instinct. Your first impression is usually right. If you don't like the outside of the office, you probably will be unhappy with what's on the inside. If the office gives you a good feeling, then more than likely, you will be pleased with the medical care.

Upon entering the office, you should be greeted by a smiling face. This will be your first face-to-face contact with the office personnel. It should be a pleasant and professional interaction. Hopefully, you came prepared for this encounter. You should be "armed" with your insurance card, your driver's license, your co-pay, and any previous medical records. You should have also completed all of the medical forms that the office requires. The forms should be the routine patient information, address, phone numbers, and contacts. There should also be a medical questionnaire that needs to be completed. In addition, the office should provide you with a HIPAA form for you to sign, a "signature on file" form so that the office can be paid for the services provided. It is also required by law that you sign an advanced directive - that is, your desires for end-of-life care and who has a power-of-attorney for you (think Terri Schiavo).

These forms are cumbersome and take time. They can be a nuisance to complete and that is why I suggest you do them in advance. It is so helpful if you bring the medical records with you. So many times, I am left in the dark as to what type of surgery or testing has been done on a patient. I will have to wait for previous medical records to arrive, before I can institute any type of treatment. That delay can be very frustrating and can have an impact on your health care. It is also helpful if you actually bring your pills with you, in their bottles from the pharmacy. It makes me crazy when a patient tells me they take a "blue pill for something". This will make it easier for the doctor to confirm your medications, doses, and your new prescription needs.

When you check in with the receptionist, ask her if the doctor is on time and schedule. You may ask how long the wait will be. Nobody likes to sit in room and wait - even if it is a "waiting" room. If the doctor is running late, you may consider re-scheduling for another appointment, or going out for something to eat or drink. If you have a good book, it can be some leisure time to catch up on some reading. However, you should be made aware of how long you can expect to wait and if the appointments usually run on schedule. Find a chair to sit in that will be comfortable for you. The chairs should be sturdy and easy to get out of. There should be plenty of magazines and maybe even a movie playing for the patients. If Jerry Springer is on and it offends you, this may be the wrong office for you. You are still in the search mode and can back out at any time. Try to find a seat alone and away from other patients. If someone has a hacking cough, you may wish to wait outside. I try to place medical masks on patients that come in with respiratory ailments. This is to prevent other patients and the staff from becoming ill.

When you are brought back to see the Physician, a nurse should have greeted you. She should take your weight, height, and vital signs (blood pressure, temperature, respiratory rate, and pulse). You should be placed in a freshly laundered or disposable gown and placed on a clean exam table. There should be disposable paper (butcher paper) covering the exam table. The nurse should obtain a brief history and take the previous medical records to make a copy, for the office file. I usually ask the nurses to obtain a brief medical history and place it in the chart. An electrocardiogram, breathing test (Spirometry), chest x-ray, and other minor tests may be performed prior to the arrival of the doctor into the exam room. For instance, if you have been a smoker for twenty years, you will need a chest x-ray.

464

6464

Upon the arrival of the Physician into the room, you will go on high alert. The doctor should be clean, professional, and offer to shake your hand. Check the doctor's shoes - if they are scuffed and tattered - beware. Sherlock Holmes said, "to check someone's shoes to look into their personality." It is not the eyes, but the shoes that are the windows into the soul.

The doctor should speak perfect English or be able to communicate in your native language. You should expect the doctor to be wearing a clean lab coat, have a stethoscope, and other doctor "stuff". You should be looked into the eyes and greeted warmly.

Do not expect to have all of your questions answered at this visit. This office visit is basically to become established with this particular Physician. You should decide whether you wish to continue to see this doctor or to continue to look around. Does this doctor meet all of your needs? Was the examination thorough? Were the appropriate questions asked and were your records reviewed? The doctor may wish to order some tests and that would be appropriate. Do not expect to have everything you need to be performed at this visit. A smart doctor will order the most expedient testing first. For example, if you are concerned about a lump on the breast, a mammogram should be the first order of business. If you have experienced some chest discomfort, an EKG, stress test and some lab work, should be done as soon as possible. Do not expect to get all of your tests ordered at this visit. This should just be the first of several office visits.

What should you expect to get done? The doctor should perform a basic physical exam. Your previous medical records and history should be reviewed. Any distressing or major concerns should be evaluated and treated at this time. You should have lab studies done (or ordered). This should include a Complete Blood Count (CBC), a SMAC-12, that is chemistries that reveal your liver, kidneys and electrolytes (Sodium and Potassium and others). You should also have a lipid profile done. This will include a cholesterol and triglyceride level, HDL, LDL, and ratios. A man over the age of 40 should have a PSA - the Prostate Blood test. A patient asked me "What kind of digital test do you use for a Prostate test"? I held up my first finger and showed it to him.

Should a rectal and pelvic exam be performed on the first visit? I don't think that is necessary to be done right away, unless you are having a specific problem related to those areas of the body. The rectal, pelvic, or genitalia exam can be done during a Sigmoidoscopy or a colonoscopy, at a later date. Unless you are having anorectal complaints as the most immediate issue, the rectal exam can be done at a later time. It is uncomfortable, embarrassing, and can make the initial office visit an unpleasant experience. Likewise, a Pap smear and breast exam should be done on a separate visit. Female health problems should be addressed and completed on a separate office visit. Most women will prefer to have this performed by their gynecologist. However, your Primary Care Physician (PCP) could certainly perform the routine female exam.

You should leave the office with orders for lab testing, and a follow-up visit. You can consider getting all of your testing ordered prior to leaving the office. This should include a chest x-ray, stress testing for heart evaluation, a Sigmoidoscopy or colonoscopy, and any referrals to specialists that you might need. These can also be received at subsequent office visits. Women should make certain that a mammogram and Pap smear have been requested.

Prior to leaving the office, you have to know this Physician's protocol for after-hours emergencies. Does the doctor take their own calls or do they share after-hours phone calls. Is there an answering service? What happens if you go to the ER during the night - who will see you?

The first office visit can be very rewarding and informative but also quite daunting. You must come prepared and don't expect everything to be done at this visit.

Truth and Reality

The Physician has to see a large number of patients every day. New patients are more difficult because of the time required to see the patient. Records have to be reviewed, exams done and tests ordered. It is so helpful for a Physician if you bring your previous medical records and medications. If the forms are completed to the best of your ability, it will also help the exam go smoother. There is nothing that frustrates me more, than a patient that refuses to complete the forms, has no records, and wants everything all at once. This is unfair and will cause a patient - Physician problem. The doctor will have to wait for previous records and this can take time and delay your medical care. Be your own advocate and come to the first visit prepared.

Summary

Make certain that the location of the office is right for you. The location as well as the appearance of the office is important. In addition, parking should be available and near the office.

The office staff should be friendly and efficient and the phones should be answered promptly.

Bring all of your medical records, prescription bottles, and completed forms with you to the first office visit.

Greet the Physician and be friendly. This is someone who will be very important in your life and you want to have a good rapport. Be supportive and respectful to the doctor. If a patient is nice and complimentary to my staff and me I will go out of my way for the patient. This is basic human nature. If I see a grumpy patient coming in, I try to spend as little time with that patient as possible. Get all of the tests ordered that you might want. If the office can't get them all done at once, ask if they can mail the test orders to you. Don't forget, the office staff will probably have to contact your insurer to obtain a referral for any ordered tests. This may take some time and effort.

Find out about after-hours emergencies. Whom do you have to contact to get care during the weekends or nights? It can't hurt to send a thank-you card to the office if they went out of their way for you.

Final Comments

I hope you have enjoyed reading this book and found it helpful. This book will help you to obtain the best medical treatment and care. Hopefully, I have explained some things that were previously confusing. Knowledge is the best way to overcome fears and to help you get the best medical care.

I have included evaluations of patients that I have treated. All of the names have been changed and all of the stories are fictional. Any resemblance to any of my patients is purely coincidental.

I would like to include more evaluations of different patients with many different types of illnesses. This will be dealt with further in a future book. You should find it helpful to see how patients are evaluated and treated, from the Physicians perspective. My next book will be out soon and is titled " So, You Want to Live Longer and Stay Healthy."

Thank you again for taking the time to read this book.

Sincerely,

Charles Lebowitz, MD, FACP

Fellow of the American College of Physicians

www.ingramcontent.com/pod-product-compliance
Lightning Source LLC
Chambersburg PA
CBHW031120180526
45160CB00005B/40/J